Nutrition and Your Life – An Unconventional Practical Approach

Nilanjana Krishnan

Valentin Razmov, Ph.D.

September 2017

Credits:
Front cover design: Stani Vlasseva
Front cover image: Hannu Viitanen (www.123rf.com/profile_anterovium)
Nilanjana Krishnan's photo: Venkatesh Kaliappan
Valentin Razmov's photo: Stani Vlasseva

Disclaimer:
The material in "Nutrition and Your Life – An Unconventional Practical Approach" is provided for educational and informational purposes only. It is not intended as medical advice. The information contained herein should not be used to diagnose or treat any illness, disease, or health condition. Use of the suggestions and information in this handbook is at the sole choice and risk of the reader.

'Nutrition and Your Life' is dense with valuable information about how we can care for ourselves and our families through healthful eating. The authors have drawn from ancient wisdom and modern science to answer many essential questions, not only about what to eat, but also how to eat for long-term health. I feel it is our responsibility, as parents, to be informed about how to nourish our families and create a foundation of self-healing for our children. This guide is an excellent, comprehensive resource to support parents in accomplishing just that. I respect and trust the wisdom that is shared in these pages, and would not hesitate to recommend this book to anyone who is ready to take responsibility for their health, and wanting practical guidance.

Kael Balizer,
Ayurvedic Practitioner
www.AyurvedaSeattle.com

Life in the modern times is anything but natural. For centuries, European and American cultures have pushed forward Man vs. Nature doctrines with the ('divine') purpose of conquering Nature and natives. The hallmarks of progress in civilization and science have often been discoveries of natural phenomena (e.g., in physics and chemistry), harnessed to 'better' our lives.

In reality, all along we have been breaking our intimate bonds with the natural world, and dislodging our habits from natural cycles. We no longer have roots of health; no recognizable stars to navigate a healthful life course. Instead, we are told what is healthy by lab scientists, government officials, and corporate salespeople. Mixed into this confusion are also voices of self-made food gurus touting numerous 'natural' diets.

'Nutrition and Your Life' by Krishnan and Razmov encourages the reader to ask basic questions, to think common sense thoughts about what food is and what your body needs. It is not preachy or dogmatic. This book helps awaken the common sensibilities within us, and gently dares us to question whether the 'plastic' foods sold to the masses are really food at all, and whether they really make us feel good. It goads us to remember deep inside what eating naturally used to be like.

As a long-time practitioner of Chinese herbal and acupuncture medicine, I daily vet questions regarding optimal foods to eat. I see patients who have terrible diets, 'unconscious' diets, or are simply confused about diets. I will recommend this excellent book to them. It will start them thinking about their food habits, and provide detailed practical information to set them on a path to develop their own optimal diet. I also recommend this book to anyone who has had nagging health problems that never have been resolved, to those who are curious about food choices but don't know whom to ask or where to start, and to those who have tried many diets and simply need to re-root themselves in common sense.

All lifestyle choices are personal, especially food. This book is a great place to start figuring out how and where to make those personal choices.

Daniel L Altschuler, Ph.D., EAMP
Clinic Director
Open Hands Medicine, Executive Director
Core faculty at Seattle Institute of Oriental Medicine (SIOM)
Adjunct faculty at Bastyr University
Seattle, Washington
www.OldSchoolAcupuncture.com
www.OpenHandsMedicine.org

Dedication

To the truth seeker that each one of us carries inside.
May you discover sustainable health and wellbeing for yourself and
your loved ones!

Acknowledgments

This handbook is the product of continued inspiration flowing from our teachers, both modern and ancient, who have passed on their timeless wisdom to us: via their own written and spoken word, as well as via the traditions and schools they have started.

We also gratefully acknowledge the support and assistance of our many friends and clients who have aided in shaping this message, so that it can become even more effective at reaching wider audiences and helping many more seekers in our world.

Our special gratitude goes to Stani Vlasseva for her thorough and invaluable feedback on versions of the manuscript, as well as for her hands-on help with the cover design. Venkatesh Kaliappan offered keen strategic insights at key points of the writing and editing process. Vladimir Ivanov helped in the final stages of putting together the book covers, and also provided specific constructive feedback on some of the content. The faculty at the Institute for Integrative Nutrition (IIN) have continually offered deep and balanced perspectives on the often polarized subjects discussed as part of this material. Finally, our families have generously and patiently provided us with the much needed mental space for this work to come to fruition.

We are grateful to all!

Contents

Foreword

I love food and everything associated; socializing, cooking, celebrations, family traditions… I love to read and learn about food and how it relates to our health and sense of wellbeing in the world. Still there are times where I find myself becoming confused about how to navigate through all the information that is out there. In our information era it can be quite overwhelming! So many people offer their opinions and emphatically tell you how to approach nutrition. It's enough to make your head spin.

What Nilanjana and Valentin offer in this handbook is a very organized guide to comprehending this topic. As you read and practice the material, you will be in a good conversation with people who have deep insights to share, and who have brought it down to earth to genuinely help you develop *your own compass and confidence*. This guide brings light to many questions that float around us, but not in a way that makes you feel as though you have only one right path to take. Nilanjana and Valentin show you that you need to tune in to yourself, and connect to your body's innate wisdom above all else. They carefully balance information with wisdom in a way that is accessible. Long before you have read to the end you will have new ideas to try in your life that are both fun and inspiring.

In my work as a child psychotherapist I am very aware of how important nutrition is to our mental wellness too. When I meet with parents and hear how anxious or depressed their child feels, I can often guess what the child's regular diet consists of. I also know how much work it is to even consider moving away from the convenience of processed foods. This handbook will offer you a way to begin to think about that in the context of your life.

What I find truly inspiring is how the authors have managed to make things accessible to all: from someone who is struggling to conceptualize potential shifts in his own nutrition to someone who has spent time studying, and even practicing, the ideas yet still needs to re-focus and find clarity about which direction to take.

May this work empower you to re-discover your own inner wisdom and deep sense of wellbeing!

Jennifer Stoakes, LMHC, Child Psychotherapist
www.PsychotherapyNW.net
June 2017
Seattle, Washington

Introduction

You may have heard experts claim: "*You are what you eat.*" What they mean is that the foods we consume are building blocks. Foods literally *become part* of our physical bodies. As food is digested, part of it is converted into biochemical energy (famously measured in calories), another part is purposed to build the cells and organs of our bodies, and a part becomes waste and is excreted as it is no longer usable by the body. Hence, the quality of the foods we choose to take in determines the qualities (i.e., healthfulness, longevity, agility, etc.) of the physical bodies we live in, and thus affects the quality of our lives.

Throughout this text we offer you fundamental principles and practices to help you make wise and empowered choices about your nutrition ("you are *what* you eat") and your life. This includes practical – yet often not widely known or shared – advice on everyday dilemmas concerning: how to make food choices that are good for you; how to deconstruct conflicting nutrition theories and dietary guidelines; how to interpret your body's signals; how to make positive shifts in your diet; how to nourish yourself beyond food; and so on. Taking a step even further, we shed light on the significance of good digestion ("you are what you *do* with what you eat") and mindful eating ("you are *how* you eat") as commonly overlooked major contributors to your lifelong wellbeing.

How is this handbook organized?
In a Q&A format, intended to break down barriers by simulating informal, friendly discussion and coaching[1], we aim to illuminate some of your most pressing questions regarding food and nutrition, and how they relate to your overall wellbeing. The flow of the writing permits reading the sections of this book in any order depending on what your personal interest and current needs are.

---

[1] A question has power in that it creates an opening for an answer to be received. Without a well-placed question, the intended recipient may not be ready to receive any answer. [Intro.1]

We begin by explaining the *unique context of modern nutrition* – and why some answers today may justifiably differ from those from a few generations ago. More than just which foods to choose (and which to avoid) for good health – although that certainly matters, too – you need to understand how the food production processes and the industry that has grown to support them may subtly influence your choices.

Having set the stage properly, we then discuss *key principles of modern nutrition*, and dive into *specific practical advice* to help you navigate the maze of options on your path toward vibrant health and optimal wellbeing. This includes a discussion of essential foods for reaching and maintaining good health; foods to be avoided; potential issues lurking behind the regular consumption of gluten, dairy, and low-fat foods, and how and where to find good quality foods. We also address thorny balancing questions like where to draw the line on sugars, how much meat is too much, how much of your food needs to be cooked versus raw, what quantity of food is beneficial to consume and how often, and many more. Some of these questions highlight the importance of an *individualized approach* to truly address *your* specific needs.

The last third of the handbook deals with the broader context of *how your food choices affect and are affected by other aspects of your life* – your habits, emotions, the people who surround you (including children who look up to you), how to prioritize changes you make to your diet, and more.

Included at the end of each question is a suggested *quick-to-implement action step* to help you integrate into your life the main ideas that have been discussed. The suggested duration of each action step is intentionally kept short, up to a few days, in order to allow you to "dip your feet" yet experience some positive change and reflect on it. When you wish to dive deeper, you can also find our second *practical suggestion with an added challenge* to help you understand the subject even better.

If your interest is kindled regarding a particular topic, you will find that we have listed several resources in §26 to help you explore subjects in greater depth. We also offer additional links to websites and other sources (books, audios, lectures) in the "References" section.

Whom is this book written for?
This material is intended for individuals and families who could relate to any of the following:

- having unsuccessfully tried to tackle a health challenge or to make a positive change related to nutrition, and now seeking practical, even unconventional, alternatives;

- espousing the motto *"an ounce of prevention is worth a pound of cure,"* or being curious to discover what such an approach could bring into their lives;

- being fairly knowledgeable on mainstream nutrition topics, and also being open to learning more about holistic ideas for living optimally;

- feeling skeptical about the value of good nutrition.

No prior knowledge of nutrition is necessary to fully understand the ideas offered here.

How does our approach differ from others on similar topics?
In the text and in many of the nearly 150 references we offer for additional exploration, you can find explanations of *the 'why'* behind the 'what' and 'how' – a valuable feature not commonly found in many publications.

In our consciously balanced and accessible presentation, *clear of dogma*, we go in depth beyond the level of typical nutrition articles and beyond conventional nutrition science. Here you will find *less well known* (or often ignored) pros and cons of various food options, as well as practical *holistic approaches*. Resting on *powerful and timeless principles* that govern good nutrition, the information is laid out so that you can be empowered to make wise choices with confidence *in your own specific situation or context* – not having to rely on generic advice and prescriptions that may not apply well (or at all) to your individual situation. (Just as a Ferrari vehicle cannot receive proper specialized service at a Toyota service station, your unique body will not be honored properly by seeking generic treatment for a specialized condition.) Yet the modern so called "health care" system does just that – offering different people the exact same treatment for a given diagnosis. We believe that the time is ripe to approach health and healing once again in a more *personalized* way – this is the fundamental frame of reference upon which our whole work is founded.

This book also stands out from many others by not limiting the discussion solely to aspects of the physical body. It incorporates *the impact of emotions, mind, and spirit to our health and wellbeing* too, offering a deeper holistic approach. Indeed, by taking good care of your physical body – with sound nutrition, proper exercise, etc. – you also open wider doors to better emotional, mental, and spiritual health and vibrancy.

All this gives the presented material a *lasting long-term value* for you.

How to use this handbook?
Integrating reading material that contains facts, anecdotes, and practical suggestions all at once can sometimes feel like a daunting task. Therefore, we invite you to pace yourself as you take in the information and implement the suggestions. We also encourage you to re-read all or portions of the material periodically, as that will help you to absorb and understand concepts that you may not have previously captured fully. A sustained focus on the concepts contained herein would be well worth the payoff – in time, money, and improved health. You and the people in your family would feel more balanced and happier.

Our intention with this work is *to empower you to take charge of your health and your life* through enhanced knowledge, body awareness, practical techniques, and conscious choices. We aim to enable you to see the bigger picture of interrelationships – between health and nutrition, and many other seemingly unrelated aspects of life. From a place of empowerment you would become an effective role model for the people around you, including children.

To make it as *personally meaningful* as possible to your loved ones, and especially to children around you, we encourage you to share the information (or its most relevant pieces) in the spirit and language most suited for their individual understanding.

How to provide feedback and further be in touch with us?
The authors are grateful for your attention, and invite your feedback and further questions to help move this valuable conversation forward – for the benefit of you and for many future readers.

You are welcome to contact us at
NutritionAndYourLife@gmail.com, as well as personally at:
HealthCoachNilanjana@gmail.com and **VRazmov@gmail.com**, respectively.

For future updates, blog articles, and communication with us, please also visit:
www.WellnessWithNilanjana.com and
www.facebook.com/nilanjana.krishnan, as well as
www.LinkedIn.com/in/VRazmov.

Part I:

A Proper Context of Modern Nutrition

1: Why do I need to know more about food and nutrition than what I already understand?

How would you feel setting foot in your world today without being able to speak, read, or write in the language that is predominantly used in your society? We all know that basic language skills are crucial to functioning effectively in our environments. Similarly, understanding the basics of how to correctly calculate payment in a store, negotiate a paycheck, or manage a credit card are essential skills for navigating our present day world well – even if you (or your child) have little interest in math. Computer literacy has lately become yet another essential skill due to the prevalence of services and jobs that require it.

Just as basic language, math, and computer literacy are now deemed fundamental requirements (not just an option) for successfully navigating in society, *nutrition-related knowledge* can also be considered fundamental and not an option – in order to do well in the world. "Why so?" you may ask.

The drastic changes to our food supply (since your grandparents' days) have been identified by scientists as a primary reason for the failing health of many people today. So learning a bit about food and nutrition – and their connection to optimal wellbeing – can make the difference for you in attaining and maintaining good health and prosperity in a world where many consume foods unknowingly and mindlessly.

You may further inquire, "I agree, times have changed and so have my eating habits, but do I still need to learn more about food and nutrition than what I already understand? Why?"

Nutrition is a fledgling science, and each day new research comes out that may dispel currently held beliefs about nutrition and health – beliefs that had been previously accepted without questioning. Therefore, it becomes increasingly and vitally important to be able to *differentiate fact from fiction* – not blindly adopting new ideas, but rather *using your own discernment* through personal experience, and determining what best serves your *individual needs*. Just as "one size does not fit all" (you may have heard the adage, "One man's food is another man's poison"), understanding and applying personalized nutrition is crucial for sustaining long-term health and wellbeing.

Furthermore, these new frontiers of nutrition-based ideas are not all founded in unbiased science. Some of the research has been funded by corporations with vested interests in swaying your opinion to serve their bottom line, often without regard to your wellbeing. Hence, the results of some nutrition and diet research may be skewed and the advice questionable. Just as adequate understanding of how financial institutions and the Internet work puts you in a better position to avoid scams in finance and online, you will – with sound knowledge of nutrition and its context in the food industry – be empowered to detect impostors in the health and nutrition-related world as well. It is therefore imperative to not only acquire basic knowledge of nutrition to apply to your daily needs, but also to cultivate the drive to *ask the right questions* to the people and institutions who are influential in the field of food production, food distribution, and general nutrition.

~

One small action step you can take today: What subject related to nutrition have you been curious about, but never really ventured to explore? Over the next week, read an article or two about it, and reflect on how that subject has evolved over the years. Has your own health or lifestyle been influenced as a result? Has your view on this subject changed over time? If yes, how?

Need an added challenge? Think of a pressing question or doubt you have regarding the efficacy of a particular product (food or non-food). Contact (call or write to) the respective authorities (e.g., manufacturer, government official, etc.) to report your concern and seek clarification. Reflect on your experience. Did you receive a prompt and satisfactory response? Did your opinion on the particular product shift as a result?

2: Whom do I trust with respect to what I should eat to be healthy? What are some good sources and practical skills?

Did you know that your body "talks" to you constantly? Your belly growls when you are hungry; you yawn when you are sleepy; when you eat too many sweets, your body craves salty foods; when you eat too much, one extra bite can make you feel nauseous; if you eat something that you are allergic to, your body may break into hives. The list goes on.

When you eat nutrient-rich foods, you feel satisfied – your mood is better and you feel good about your choices. These are some of the ways your body tells you that it is happy. On the other hand, if you eat junk foods, you will often find yourself hungry very soon, low on energy, and lethargic, wishing you had made better choices, and your body craving real, nutritious foods. Unfortunately, many people misunderstand or ignore that signal and give more of the same nutrient-deficient foods to the body, perpetuating this cycle. Yes, your body gives you constant feedback, and nobody can understand your body better than you.

Once upon a time, man could eat foods growing in the wild. Based on how it tasted and smelled, he could discern if it was nourishment or poison. However, you cannot do the same in the modern world since many foods have been specifically engineered – by man, not by Nature[2] – to appeal to your taste buds, even though in reality they may be devoid of any nutrition whatsoever. As a result, taste has become an invalid means to discern healthy from unhealthy foods. Thus, it is important to upgrade your knowledge about the health qualities of the foods you normally consume and prefer. [2.1, 2.2, 2.3]

You have the privilege of choosing what to eat and what to avoid. The key to your wellbeing lies with you! So empower yourself to stay informed, and trust yourself to make responsible choices. If you are

---

[2] Here and subsequently "Nature" (with a capitalized "N") refers to "Mother Nature," whereas "nature" (with a lowercase "n") refers to a person's innate nature.

just starting on this journey, treat it as a path of (re)discovery. Make hypotheses, experiment, observe results, analyze the results, and iterate – integrating your deeper understanding and greater confidence over time.

Here are *specific techniques* to help you listen to your body's cues and feedback more clearly:

Technique	Explanation
Take three deep, conscious breaths	Deliberately introduces a pause before you dive into your plate (or before any other action). Allows you to prepare your body to receive the desired nourishment. Gives you a moment to cast your eyes on the lovely spread before you. Also nourishes you on many levels – visually, emotionally – and contributes to your overall sense of satisfaction from (even less) food.
Consciously slow down and eat mindfully	Chew carefully and take the time to breathe deeply. Go at a pace where you can be aware of the specific foods you put into your mouth. Take the time to taste the various foods. Allow yourself to be fully present with the food while eating – the key is where your focus lies. This nourishes you physically, emotionally, and mentally. [2.4] Above all, start small – do the above for one meal each day, or for a day or two when you are not rushed.
Silently offer gratitude to the people and resources that went into bringing this nutritious food to you	Positively shifts your relationship to food – from needing or craving it to simply appreciating food for the sustenance it provides to you. Better aligns your own energies with those of the food you are consuming, thereby improving absorption. In turn, this creates positive changes in your body, and moves you toward physical wellbeing. [2.4, 2.5]

Technique	Explanation
Muscle test[3] – to obtain a "yes" or "no" answer to questions you pose	Allows you to decipher if a specific food (or exercise, person, habit, thought, or idea in question) is well suited for you in the present moment. This is based on how your muscles strengthen or weaken in response to a specific input from you: a question you pose, an object you hold close, or a thought you focus on.
Silently communicate directly with your body	Pose a question silently, then intently and intuitively sense your body's response (e.g., tightening of stomach muscles, lightness around the heart, etc.) to it. Similarly to the muscle testing technique (above), this can be used to seek input from your body (e.g., on a food-related question).

Regularly putting to practice these simple techniques will help you to pay closer attention to your body in the present moment: how it feels, what it needs. As you become seasoned in this process of tuning within and deciphering your body's signals, you will be able to expand your awareness to your emotional states of mind too: whether you are upset, angry, sad, joyful, contented, excited. Once you develop and maintain keen awareness of your physical and emotional states, you will feel empowered to make your own appropriate choices that help you to attain and sustain a steadier state of wellbeing.

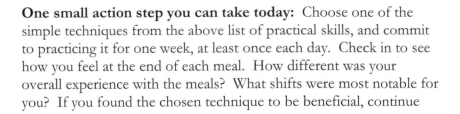

One small action step you can take today: Choose one of the simple techniques from the above list of practical skills, and commit to practicing it for one week, at least once each day. Check in to see how you feel at the end of each meal. How different was your overall experience with the meals? What shifts were most notable for you? If you found the chosen technique to be beneficial, continue

---

[3] Applied kinesiology uses self-driven or aided muscle-testing techniques to obtain "yes" or "no" answers from your energy field, as dictated by your subconscious mind. [2.6, 2.7, 2.8, 2.9]

doing it regularly for another three weeks – this additional practice time will transform it into "second nature" for you!

Need an added challenge? Practice all the above listed techniques for 4 weeks. Keep track in a journal of what you have learned and experimented with along the way. Reflect upon your new abilities of tuning within. What new aspects of your body – physical, mental, and emotional – are being revealed to you?

3: What does a healthy choice mean?

As children grow up, they naturally face an increasing number of possibilities in the world around them. So they often hear general advice such as "Make a wise choice." To correctly interpret and act on such advice, it is important to know – both for parents and children – what "wise" means in each specific context.

When it comes to food and nutrition, a synonymous term would be "healthy." So let us first define what constitutes a *"healthy choice."* Thus we will lay the groundwork for some of the following discussion in this handbook. Subsequent questions will then dive deeper into the individual concepts and practices. Here it is worth mentioning that just because some food product may have the word "healthy" on its packaging does not yet mean that the claim is true – one has to look deeper, including by reading labels.

Borrowing from time-honored wisdom in other disciplines, in order to properly define something a set of key questions need to be answered first, namely: *who, where, when, what, why, how,* and *how much.* This is known as the W^5H^2 model [3.1] (following the first letter of each of these seven constitutive questions).

To apply this model to our case, the definition of a "healthy choice" will correspondingly depend on: *who* you are, *where* you are, *when* you eat, *what* you eat, *why* you eat, *how* you eat, and *how much* you eat. Let us briefly explain.

***Who* you are:** On a personal level, this implies your *individual constitution*, i.e., your age, body type[4], blood type, activity level, etc. What is healthy *for you* could differ depending on each of those aspects. While there are general guidelines (discussed later) that apply to most people seeking to attain health, there is no "one-size-fits-all" when it comes to tuning your own system well.

On a different dimension, *who you are* implies your role in the larger connected world around you. If you are a parent or an adult, you

---

[4] To find out your individual body type, refer to the references for §5.

naturally serve as a model for children around you, whether or not this is your goal. So being mindful of your *context* and acting in ways that are thoughtful, conscious, and deliberate can help to instill a similar attitude in growing children, serving them well for a lifetime. This handbook is specifically designed to help guide you toward such thoughtful, conscious, and deliberate choices in food and nutrition.

Where **you are:** Your location in the world determines more than just where you physically are at a given time. It determines what food choices may be available in your surroundings. Do you live in a place that features regular Farmers' Markets, or do you live in a "food desert" with only a few convenience stores selling mostly packaged processed foods? Do you eat mostly at home, or do you eat out often? What does the prevalent culture around you dictate when it comes to food? Some of these food choices may be quite new to you, making it harder to tell which of them may be decent options. Some may not be optimal according to your understanding, yet you still need to make regular wise choices from whatever is available.

If you cook at home, be mindful of the ingredients you put into meals, including sauces, flavorings, etc. It matters what their origin is, and whether there are any "impostors" among them. Similarly, if you eat out at a restaurant, as much as possible pick dishes that imply the presence of healthful ingredients and minimize those which do not. If you are frequently traveling for extended periods of time, build a habit of eating when you can be calm and stationed (e.g., not in a moving vehicle). Above all, apply common sense – it is often best to answer genuine hunger cues from your body than to ignore them repeatedly for lack of a "proper" environment. Details about much of this will follow on subsequent pages.

When **you eat:** The body processes food differently depending on the time of day (or night)[5]. Not all times are equally effective. People have developed habits of eating at certain times, often based on the context they are surrounded by, but these may not be optimal

---

[5] The physical body also processes food differently depending on the type of food, how it has been prepared, and a number of other factors. For the purposes of the above discussion we focus on the timing aspect.

times for good assimilation of the food, and consequently for maintaining good health.

On another dimension, when food is taken in after a genuine signal from the body (for this, having good body awareness helps), the digestion and absorption will happen easier and be more complete since the body will be prepared. Conversely, if food is consumed without a physical need – e.g., because you may be feeling nervous or just sitting in front of the TV – the result will not be beneficial to your health.

***What* you eat:** The food you consume becomes partly fuel for your body's energy needs, and partly building blocks that become your future body. So it is very important what you put in – including consuming the right kinds of foods, the right quantities, and the correct combinations for *your* body. Are the ingredients whole(some) or processed? Is your diet balanced, including all major groups of macro- and micro-nutrients? These topics are elaborated on further below.

***Why* you eat:** Ideally, you would eat based on a conscious decision and self-awareness. But for many people food choices are instead determined based on many other unrelated factors. This includes: influences by people (who may not know better) and situations (e.g., school food vs. home-cooked food; children who regularly need to shift home environments due to parent separation); available discounts at local stores; marketing recommendations (e.g., "Got milk?"); available stock inside a nearby vending machine; or the implied urgency in the availability of a treat on a party platter or in a store (e.g., "Sale ends soon," "While supplies last," etc.).

The sense of hunger is a key *pre-requisite* for consuming food. Note, however, that cravings are not the same as hunger – though they are often misinterpreted that way. Cravings are instead a messenger (sent by your body) for something that is lacking in your life; they may or may not be nutrition-related. Cravings are best handled by seeking out and tackling the root causes of what is missing, rather than by simply shutting down the signal (through eating food). Scientists have shown that the sense of joy and happiness, inherently sought by all humans, is associated with the release of nitric oxide internally in the tissues of the body, while the absence of such positive emotions forces the body to obtain the nitric oxide through different means, including through the consumption of food (mostly sweets and their derivatives). [3.2] Do you really need that piece of cake, or is it just masking a lack of sweetness in your close relationships?

How you eat: As we just mentioned, your present state of mind and emotions affects how you eat. The reverse is also true – how you eat influences your mind and emotions, as well as your physical body. [3.3] In that regard, the simple mindfulness and self-awareness practices suggested previously – e.g., breathing deeply, eating slowly, paying attention to each bite, chewing well, putting yourself in a calm environment and a peaceful state of mind, being grateful for the food you have – can all help you to establish and sustain a sound basis for overall health and wellbeing.

Conversely, if you eat under stress, many of the natural feedback signals that your body utilizes to communicate to you get suppressed and may be easily missed or ignored. Reflecting on your own experience, is it the case that the times when you have overeaten in the past were situations when you were not consciously aware and fully present? Perhaps you were under some type of stress?

How much you eat: Portion size matters. Meal frequency matters. Even if you take in an otherwise healthy food, too much or too little cannot be a path to wellness. How much is appropriate for you depends in turn on *who you are*: on your individual constitution (i.e., stage in life, body type and size, activity level, etc.). Hence, an individualized approach is imperative.

For best results, controlling the quantity and frequency of your meals must be a *conscious process*. It gets better with experience and with developed self-awareness (including body awareness) and focus.

In the remaining pages you will learn much more about all of these topics.

Finally, in order to truly make healthy choices, one must look beyond the 'I' and consider which choices are *healthy and sustainable for our collective environment* too. We are all interdependent with everyone and everything else, and our individual choices and actions create ripple effects in the whole. Each one of us is a tiny yet significant slice of the world "pie," influencing neighboring slices and making a difference. Whether we tend to our world on a microscopic level (i.e., caring for individual beings and their immediate environment) or a macroscopic level (i.e., caring for the world as a whole), the results ultimately come to affect all. The gentle care we like to apply toward ourselves must extend out and include all else also.

$\sim$

One small action step you can take today: Look at the W^5H^2 model described above. Select at least one of the "W" and "H" factors, and see how they fit and/or describe you, your lifestyle, and your environment. Do your eating habits line up with what you identified as a result of this exercise? If yes, how? If not, what would it take for you to make the necessary shift(s)?

Need an added challenge? Based on the same W^5H^2 model, select one aspect under each "W" and "H." Then map them out to see how it describes you, your lifestyle, and your environment. Now consider how your choices may be impacting your individual environment (e.g., family) and your collective environment (e.g., community, planet). Do you feel inspired to make any changes? If yes, how?

4: How come my parents / grandparents / ancestors ate not the way we are advised to, yet still lived "fine"? What has gone wrong since?

A bygone era remembered

The environment in which our ancestors lived had little resemblance to what we have today. There was more biodiversity and the land / soil was naturally fertile, hence more conducive to cultivating healthy crops sustainably. Life moved at a slower, more comfortable pace. People spent time making home-cooked meals each day, while outside food and restaurant visits were reserved for special events and celebrations. Food was ingested to provide nutrition for sustenance and to stave off hunger. The air, water, food, and environment in general were cleaner and more pristine, with hardly any toxic elements injected by industrial operations. Children played outside in the dirt, not with technology gadgets, so a deeper personal connection with Mother Earth and a reverence for Nature was cultivated.

A contrasting picture of Now

In recent years, food throughout much of the world has increasingly become an article of entitlement, status, and identity, even used as entertainment to ward off boredom, loneliness, and emotional disturbances. Modern day people often eat (or snack) whether or not they are truly hungry, hence confusing their body systems. The "convenience" of prepared foods has caused more inconvenience in the end – leading many people out of their home kitchens and into grocery stores' prepared foods sections or into fast food pick-up lanes, thereby leading to reliance on poor quality foods. People seem to rush about everywhere (e.g., at work, in schools). Many choose to inundate themselves with much "stuff": fast cars, a variety of electronic devices, and much more. Our environment, too, has progressively degraded due to uncontrolled toxic emissions, industrial agriculture, rampant use of synthetic chemical fertilizers and pesticides, and genetically engineered crops. At the same time, people's level of activity has changed much – in the old days physical activity was dominant, while nowadays there is much sitting still in one place, leading to decreased exercising of the physical bodies.

Thus, stressors of all kinds – physical, mental, emotional, social, and environmental – have become much more prevalent in modern life.

The face of modern food production

Today's industrialized, conventional food production is less and less about sound agricultural practices. Instead, it has become an enormous and influential industry, with economic incentives favoring companies that produce low-cost foods and often make misleading claims about the health-related qualities of such foods. Food packaging features enticing words such as "natural," "healthy," and "clean" – yet the use of these words is often not regulated, so the claims may be entirely untrue. Additionally, just because a food may contain some percentage of, say, "whole" grains on the ingredients list does not yet mean that the food *as a whole* is healthful. [4.1]

Artificial homogenization within the food industry

In most developed (and developing) countries today, the concept of supermarkets is not only popular but also a widely accepted channel for delivering all sorts of items (food and non-food) that people may desire. However, up until a few decades ago, the idea of a supermarket was foreign to people. They commonly relied on their local and neighborhood grocer or farm stand for their food-related needs, and on other general or specialty stores for non-food items. In those days, it was rare to find a "super store" catering to your every need, from food to toothpaste to AA batteries to paper plates to toilet paper! There are advantages to having all your needs met under one roof: making a one-stop shop may save you time and energy (and perhaps even gasoline). However, today's supermarkets carry more or less the same kinds and brands of products, creating a highly homogeneous marketplace of "more of the same."
Items commonly available in small, family-owned shops are often unique and non-homogeneous, but supermarkets do not generally carry them either because relatively smaller manufacturers are unable to match the scale of production desired by large stores or the items are not as price competitive.

Over time, this has resulted in an environment of "artificial homogenization" of products, and has placed customers like you in the grip of large stores and manufacturers. The market has become monopolized by few (food and non-food related) manufacturing companies that are more focused on improving their bottom lines, and less on enhancing your life. Due to heavy competition and the desire to make their products appear prominently on store shelves, such manufacturers also lower their prices by compromising on both the quality of their products and on the wages of their employees and suppliers (including food growers). In the end, a product you buy today at a supermarket may look somewhat like what your parents used to buy years ago, but its essence has fundamentally and invisibly deteriorated.

Marketing strategies driving compulsive behaviors

You may walk into a store with a shopping list for ten items, but may leave the store with fifteen (if not more) items. Why has this pattern become so common? Grocery stores intentionally offer more than what you really need – e.g., products on shelves at the check-out lanes; heavy discounts and/or limited-time offers (e.g., "Get 2 for the price of 1, this weekend only"). Therefore, your food (and non-food) choices often become unconsciously driven by convenience, shrewd marketing tactics, a felt sense of having made a "sound" purchasing decision, and so on. So you end up purchasing more than your own personal needs at that time. With extra "goodies" on hand, you may be inclined to alter your plans for what you will eat that day (or in the near future), in order to effectively use up the extra food products / ingredients you have purchased. For example, you may have planned to prepare a vegetable soup that evening, but because you bought an extra pack of cheese (due to some "Buy 1, Get 1 free" offer at the store), you decide to have creamy Fettuccine Alfredo instead. Perhaps you felt compelled to use some of the cheese while still fresh, lest it gets stale or spoils soon. In the end, you consume food not so much dictated by your original intention or bodily needs, but rather by sheer compulsion.

As the evidence points out, there have been many big changes since the days of our ancestors – in the attitudes towards food, health, and buying behavior. What was once considered a necessity has today become a source of indulgence, driving compulsive behaviors.

$\sim$

One small action step you can take today: Just for a day, get into your "grandparents' shoes" (grandma's or grandpa's – you decide ☺). Look at your food choices – whether you eat at home or outside – and select only the ones with ingredients that your ancestors might recognize. How does eating this way make you feel? Are you able to locate enough food choices to satisfy your hunger? What did you learn from this experience? Although seemingly simple, this exercise may feel like a real challenge at first; yet if you choose to do this every day for 3-4 weeks, it will become "second nature" to you.

Need an added challenge? Stay in your "grandparents' shoes" for four weeks, and while you are at it practice "sticking to the list" when you go shopping (for food and/or non-food items). Resist the urge to pick up that one extra item that is not on your list. Do you feel empowered when living this way? If yes, how? If not, what do you think stands in the way? How can you overcome this situation?

Part II:

Principles and Nitty-Gritty of Nutritional Advice

5: Which foods are good for me? Do my needs change over time, and how?

There are several important principles to be aware of in choosing good foods:

Pick easily recognizable ingredients. Foods that have one ingredient or *just a few easily recognizable (and pronounceable!) ingredients* are generally among the best options to pick from. Vegetables, fruits, whole grains, nuts, and some minimally processed foods such as some forms of bread, cultured dairy products like yogurt and cheese, and good fats such as those present in coconut oil, grass-fed butter, olive oil, and avocado oil are some *generally* good options for healthy food. Still, always take your individual present situation into account, and use body awareness to guide your choices.

Honor your own individual needs. *No two people's bodies are exactly alike*, so it is important to *understand your own body* and its current needs based on age, activity level, time of the year, etc., and even based on non-obvious factors such as present health condition (chronic or acute), temporary changes in hormonal activity, etc. To truly optimize for your individual needs, it would help to know your body's constitution, as dictated by factors like blood type (based on your blood group), metabolic type (based on how your body metabolizes), Ayurvedic energy type (based on how you perform physical, mental, emotional and behavioral functions), and other relevant metrics. [5.1, 5.2, 5.3, 5.4, 5.5]

Monitor your body's reactions. Food allergies and sensitivities also influence which foods may be better for you. Hence, one way to select appropriate foods for you personally is by experimentation: first eliminating foods you consume regularly or suspect are causing you discomfort (physical or other), and then gradually reintroducing them one at a time while *monitoring your own body's reactions* all along[6].

---

[6] The exact same approach is recommended for introducing infants to solid foods – one new food item at a time, starting with small doses.

Choose a variety of wholesome foods. Pick vegetables and fruits that come in all colors of the rainbow. "Eating a rainbow" provides your body with many different nutrients, as each color comes with its own unique combination of vitamins and minerals. [5.6] As you include such a variety in your daily diet, the desire for less nutritious (and less natural) foods will gradually diminish also. You will likely start consuming less and less of those "allergenic" foods (or foods you may be sensitive to). [5.7]

Eat according to the season. It may serve you well to *align your diet with the seasons* – eating lighter (and more alkaline) foods, such as berries, cherries, jicama, celery, lemons, etc., in the warmer months; and eating heavier, richer (and more acidic) foods, such as dairy, eggs, nuts, heartier winter vegetables (e.g., pumpkin, squashes, potatoes), animal proteins, heart-healthy fats, etc., in the cooler months. Staying in tune with Nature and eating what grows (or is easily available) in your locale in a particular season is one way of receiving Nature's bounty and thus honoring your own inner nature. If people ate more seasonally and consumed fewer processed foods, most allergies and food sensitivities could be alleviated. [5.8, 5.9]

Combine raw, cooked, and juiced foods. Eating foods in various forms – *raw, cooked, or juiced* – enables you to assimilate the available nutrients differently. For example, vegetable juicing makes the nutrients and anti-oxidants more bioavailable; the cooking process removes certain acids / anti-nutrients[7], allowing access to key nutrients (e.g., beta carotene in carrots) that would otherwise be less available. However, anti-oxidants and vitamins are lost when cooking or juicing at high temperatures or for a longer time – which underscores the value of raw foods, too. This theme of raw vs. cooked foods is discussed more extensively in §9.

Overall, well-selected foods (as described), consumed in proper dosage (which in turn depends on factors such as your age, gender, activity level, specific constitution, hormonal activity, etc.) can be nourishing and beneficial for you.

---

[7] Anti-nutrients are compounds present in foods that interfere with the absorption of nutrients. They are a part of the plants' self-protective mechanisms. Examples include phytic acid, oxalates, lectins, etc.

~

One small action step you can take today: When choosing vegetables and fruits to add to your meals, pick ones of every color – white, purple, blue, green, yellow, orange, red, and more as you can find. Eat that way (combined in a single meal or spread across several meals and snacks) for three consecutive days. How do you feel on day three? If "eating a rainbow" has been beneficial to you, continue to consciously incorporate as many colors as you can (from *unprocessed and wholesome* vegetables and fruits) each day, thereby "crowding out" any highly processed and less nutritious foods from your diet.

Need an added challenge? Select just one food that you either eat in large quantities every day, or that you suspect may be causing some allergic responses or other uncomfortable symptoms in your body. Completely eliminate that particular food for one week, replacing it with wholesome alternatives of which you already eat some regularly. Notice how you begin to feel by the end of the week. Now reintroduce that food back on day eight. How do you feel? Do you have more energy or less? Based on how you feel you can determine if that food is health promoting or health depleting for you. Please note that very often when you temporarily give up foods (whether agreeable to your health or not) that you have been eating regularly, you may experience withdrawal symptoms (i.e., you may feel worse for a bit, until you start feeling better). It is recommended that you do not attempt to eliminate too many foods at a time without expert supervision.

6: Which foods are essential for a healthy life? Why?

Depending on the culture you were brought up in, you may have grown up with concepts like a food pyramid or a food plate. These are simplified, illustrative ways to communicate the main categories of recommended nutrients to include in meals for the purposes of sustaining good health.

Basic nutritional building blocks

It is broadly agreed that in order to function well the human body needs a certain amount of carbohydrates, proteins, fats, as well as vitamins and dietary fiber. These components each serve a different purpose, so more of one cannot replace or compensate for another. Some of these nutrients can be readily converted to energy that the body needs. Others make good *building blocks* for replacing cells in the body. Yet others support (i.e., catalyze, control) the digestive (metabolic) processes that define much about how the physical body works.

The importance of supplementation

It may also be good to take supplements (e.g., multivitamin, iron, omega-3, vitamin D, vitamin B_{12}, etc.), because there is no easy way to tell how many kinds of nutrients (e.g., vitamins and minerals) and how much of each nutrient are present in any given food. This is partly due to our modern-day living: few people grow their own food, while most of us rely heavily on grocery stores and/or Farmers' Markets to get food supplies. Most regular grocery stores receive a large percentage of their produce from faraway places (including national and international markets). To travel such long distances, fruits and vegetables need to be harvested much ahead of their natural ripening in order to reduce spoilage while en route. Such early harvesting results in a reduction of nutrients for the fresh produce. This situation is exacerbated when people also eat fast foods or prepared frozen foods, thereby further diminishing their total intake of real nutrients in a given day. Additionally, many of us live very differently from our ancestors and the way the human body has evolved to function. We spend much time indoors, work long hours on computers, or eat foods that are either out of season or not in accordance with our body constitution (e.g., not getting vitamin D directly from the sun; not having enough hemoglobin or ferritin reserves due to an unbalanced vegetarian diet, etc.). Hence, taking supplements is a practical way to deliver necessary nutrients to the body – nutrients, which may not otherwise be readily available through the foods due to our modern lifestyles and food production methods.

Bringing nutritional balance

What different schools sometimes disagree on is the relative percentages of nutrient components in a healthy diet. Yet almost universally acknowledged is the *principle of balance* – the notion that we need some of each of these constitutive nutrients: not too little and not too much. Similarly, it has been established that meals are absorbed best in the human body when they are neither too acidic, nor too alkaline as a whole. Hence, some practical knowledge about which foods are more acidic vs. more alkaline can be additionally helpful. [6.1]

Attitude impacts food and health

Of importance to creating a good, nutritious meal is also how the food is prepared. Part of this comes with the (positive) attitude and care taken by the cook. That is why home-prepared meals can often be more satisfying, beyond merely enhancing the taste.

Effects of different methods of food preparation

Another aspect of preparation is that cooking is preferable for certain foods, while for others it is not advisable. For example, cooking can soften the otherwise hard cell walls of carrots and asparagus or broccoli stems, thus "unlocking" (i.e., improving the digestibility of) more of the nutrients inside. The absorption can sometimes be further enhanced by the use of oils. At the same time, for many fruits and soft vegetables (e.g., salads) the process of cooking (or even juicing, if the juicer heats up by spinning too rapidly) can greatly diminish the nutritional value and destroy available vitamins. High-heat cooking (including by deep frying, char-grilling, or microwaving) is known to radically alter the properties of food ingredients, to the point of actually rendering food harmful for consumption. [6.2, 6.3] For example, certain oils and fats (if not suitable for high-heat cooking [6.4]), all meats, and even honey can be thus adversely affected.

Other methods of preparation exist that can enhance the quality of foods. Sprouting makes seeds even more potent and beneficial. Soaking for an extended period (generally, for 6-8 hours) and then peeling skins cleanses nuts of potentially harmful substances (e.g., phytic acid in peanuts). Fermenting foods (e.g., dairy to make kefir, cabbage to make sauerkraut, green tea to make Kombucha, etc.) helps to increase the beneficial gut bacteria, and the food is pre-digested, so the load on the digestive system is reduced, in turn making it easier to absorb nutrients. [6.5]

The inherent nature of food's energy serving as medicine
For a truly healthy life, not only the body but also the mind and emotions need to be well balanced. While it is widely known that proper nutrition supports a healthy body, it is also true that food affects our state of mind and emotions. The inherent energetics[8] of foods can indeed be harnessed to appropriately address specific mental and emotional imbalances. For example, if you are feeling heavy, lethargic, and lacking energy or initiative to move about or get things done, this may be balanced by eating foods that grow above the ground, such as green leafy vegetables, quinoa, corn, and certain fruits that embody the qualities of flexibility and lightness. These food plants all literally sway in the winds, creating an ease of movement, flexibility, and lightness. Conversely, if you are feeling too spacy, ungrounded, and anxious, this may be balanced by consuming more foods that grow on or below the ground, those whose quality is one of grounding, heaviness, and solidity, such as pumpkin, yam, and potato. Similarly, chicken soup is commonly given for recovery from colds, because chickens in general have the qualities of alertness, perkiness, and swiftness, precisely what a person who has a cold lacks in their body. The general principle through all these examples is to *seek within Nature the qualities that your body, mind, or emotions may be lacking.* [6.6, 6.7, 6.8]

~

---

[8] The term "energetics" refers to how energy flows or is stored in a system (e.g., a plant, a tree, a human, or any non-living entity).

One small action step you can take today: For one week, in at least one of your meals each day make sure that your plate contains a balance of vegetables, protein, grains, and fats. How is your energy level and mood after eating a balanced meal? Was your experience different from other mealtime experiences? If so, how?

Need an added challenge? For three days experiment with the various techniques for preparing vegetables that help to preserve most, if not all, of their nutrients. You may choose one or more methods such as: steaming, sautéing, baking, fermenting, sprouting, or eating raw. However, please ensure that if you cook the vegetables, the cooking temperature should remain low to medium, and you do not overcook them. Stay away from high-heat cooking such as using a microwave, char-grilling, deep-frying, or eating highly processed foods. Did you notice any difference in your energy levels when eating vegetables prepared in this manner? Which was your favorite preparation technique, and why?

7: Are there foods that are best avoided? Why?

As we have already discussed, the concept of what constitutes food to the body has evolved much. On the most basic level, food is what nourishes the physical body. Over time and in an attempt to offer new food choices and tastes, man has created and *engineered* numerous new *food-like substances* (while at the same time, sadly, diminishing the *biodiversity of natural foods[9]*), substances that lack this quality of providing proper nourishment. For many modern-day people, especially in the developed world, food has become an object of exploration, of entertainment, of addiction, even of ideology – obscuring its most fundamental essence as serving to continuously nourish the physical body.

It is therefore these *food-like substances* – not real foods – that you need to distinguish and handle properly. We refer to them as "food-like," because they often look like, taste like, or feel like natural foods, yet they are not real food and their effect on our bodies may be quite different and indeed undesirable.

Chief among food-like substances that modern people consume are two categories:

- those that are grown in unnatural conditions (e.g., using pesticides, using genetically modified seeds, etc.), and

- those that have been heavily processed ("refined," or even cooked) before consumption.

These two categories have dramatically expanded in recent decades throughout the world, generally at the cost of reduced availability and lower consumption of more natural foods, leading to a negative impact on the health of the people whose food chains and environment have been disturbed. An illustrative example is the increasing reliance on monocultures[10], driven by pressures from large

---

[9] A deep subject with significant ramifications for all life, biodiversity needs to be properly addressed in a larger body of work. It is beyond the scope of this writing.

[10] The term monoculture refers to a single crop grown repeatedly in a given area.

corporations. For example, potatoes ("Russet Burbank" variety) are intensively farmed as a monoculture crop by certain farmers in Idaho, USA to meet a burgeoning demand for French fries by the fast food giant McDonald's Corp. The company has stipulated certain metrics for the potatoes they require for their French fries recipe. To sustain such a high-yielding crop year after year, farmers have used harmful chemical fertilizers and pesticides. The result of this process of cultivating chemical-dependent monocultures is that over time: (a) the ecological balance of the land is destroyed, disrupting the natural food chains; (b) the nutrients in the food crop are reduced; and (c) harmful chemical toxins are introduced in the crop and also in the land. [7.1] Regular consumption of such highly processed toxic food contributes to an increasing trend in many illnesses.

Type of processing	Known effects
Using pesticides and insecticides on plants, administering antibiotics to animals, or cooking in pots and pans that have a non-stick surface (e.g., Teflon)	The chemical residues of these substances are harmful and have an adverse effect on human health, water quality, soil depletion, etc. [7.2, 7.3, 7.4, 7.5]
Genetic modification	The hi-tech modification process radically alters the nature of food, and comes at a cost to both human health and the environment. [7.6, 7.7, 7.8, 7.9]
Heavy food processing: adding synthetic preservatives, artificial colors and flavors, large amounts of salt, refined sugars, other stimulants	Chemicals disturb the balance of nutrients in food: the original beneficial ingredients are largely destroyed, while harmful compounds are introduced.
Heavy cooking: char-grilling, deep frying, using microwave ovens	High temperatures and ionizing radiation alter the nature of food: the original beneficial ingredients are largely destroyed, while harmful compounds are introduced.

Type of processing	Known effects
Creating alcoholic beverages	Stimulants constitute a poison to the human body on a cellular level. Especially high-% alcohols, when used in unregulated quantities, cause harm to the nervous system, spike blood sugar levels, and damage the liver.

When ignorance is not bliss

Just because most of us are not equipped to readily understand such technological processes in detail does not mean that those processes have no impact on human health. Quite the opposite – the less aware you are, the more you can become a victim of false marketing, and the less incentive there will be for food producers and processors to act ethically and responsibly in order to stay in business. Hence the importance of increasing your *conscious awareness* in the choices you make. For example, you may be keenly aware of the presence of potential allergens in a given food, because of adverse reactions you may have witnessed in yourself or others. If you then "vote with your money" and buy other foods that do not cause such problems, you will effectively give economic signals to some food manufacturers that their product is inferior, and to others that their offering is superior.

So the question becomes: is there an (easy) way to tell what (if any) processing a given food option has undergone? This is partly the subject of several upcoming questions, so read on.

Conscious consumption of "non-food" foods

More broadly, applying conscious awareness to your choices can make a positive difference for you – not only related to foods you eat, but also to other non-food factors that also "feed" you, whether or not they serve you well. For example, are your relationships nurturing or toxic? Is your career / vocation based on *your* choice or someone else's? Is your regular physical activity / exercise enjoyable or stressful? Is your spiritual practice rooted in love (hence uplifting and expansive) or fear (hence limiting and repressive)? *Conscious awareness* is the first step toward empowering you to positively transform all these aspects of your life.

~

One small action step you can take today: Scan your pantry and refrigerator. Take a closer look at what you have stocked in there. Read the ingredients list and see if you can identify any "food-like" substances among them. Were you surprised at what you uncovered? Would you be willing to replace the items containing questionable ingredients with foods that contain wholesome ingredients? If not, what is stopping you? What did you learn from this exercise about yourself and about the foods?

Need an added challenge? For one week, commit to reading product and nutrition labels. Buy and consume, as much as possible, foods made with good quality ingredients (not food impostors), grown pesticide-free, and free of genetically engineered ingredients. How do you feel at the end of the week? What shifts, if any, did you experience physically, mentally, or emotionally?

8: Is there a problem with sugary foods?

Foods can be categorized by six tastes: sweet, sour, salty, pungent, bitter, and astringent[11]. According to the science of Ayurveda, you can maintain optimum health if you incorporate all six tastes in every meal, and by adjusting the quantities of each taste, depending on your individual constitution. In the modern civilization, many people lose touch with this timeless nutrition wisdom, and consume more and more of just a few of these taste categories. Here we explore the popular sweet taste, how it has evolved over time, and how it impacts your health.

Evolution of the sweet taste

Humans are genetically predisposed to prefer sweet tastes. Sweet foods found in Nature are generally considered safe sources of energy and nutrients. In ancient times when food was scarce, humans evolved and adapted to prefer sweet foods.[12] For humans, sweetness is harder than other tastes to detect. In the natural settings where our ancestors evolved, sweetness (detectable at 1 part per 200 of sucrose in a solution) indicated energy density, while bitterness (detectable at 1 part per 2,000,000 of quinine in a solution) suggested a possible toxicity. The much lower bitterness detection threshold would have predisposed us to avoid bitter-tasting foods, while seeking out sweet-tasting (and hence energy-dense) foods. Even among leaf-eating primates, there is a tendency to prefer immature leaves, which tend to be slightly sweeter, higher in protein, and lower in poisons than more mature leaves. Humans are also "programmed" to like sweet foods because a mother's milk – the very first food most of us have taken in – is predominantly sweet and also nutrient-dense. [8.1, 8.2, 8.3, 8.4]

Fast forward to more recent times, and notice how across cultures people continue to gravitate toward sweet tasting foods. When a celebration or offering takes place, sweets are generally the preferred choice. Many people like to reward (themselves or others) with sweet treats. It is no wonder then that humans are indeed wired for the

---

[11] Recently, people have started referring to yet another taste, called umami.
[12] Sweet taste encouraged the Paleolithic man to eat more fruit, and thus he would get enough Vitamin C.

sweet taste – genetically, anthropologically, and culturally. The pervasive presence of sugar in human societies perpetuates itself easily, because sugar is highly addictive (estimated to be 8 times more addictive than even the notorious cocaine [8.5]) and can also be derived (even engineered, more recently) from many sources, available in all locales throughout the globe. Today, with the great variety of sweet foods readily available in most developed and developing countries, our innate preference for such foods has led to wide-spread and serious health-related challenges. Only recently, however, have open-minded researchers begun to "connect the dots" and understand that there is a common cause behind many modern-day ailments – the out-of-control consumption of sugars.

Sweetness vs. "sugariness"

While there is nothing inherently wrong with sweet foods, many health advocates of today demonize sweets. Why? There are several contributing factors to this. One is a drastic change in recent times that made the notion of "sweetness" become identical to "sugariness." "What is the difference?" you may ask. A ripe banana is sweet and so is a pop tart. One is inherently sweet (i.e., created by Mother Nature), whereas the other has been sweetened (i.e., created by food engineers). Traditionally, sugar has been derived from sugarcane, one of the oldest cultivated crops known to man. However, since the advent of biotechnology, genetic engineering, and food industry-funded research, several high sweetness-yielding substances have been created: high fructose corn syrup, beet sugar, maltose, dextrose, maltodextrin, saccharin, aspartame, and more. We recommend that you stay away from all of these! While it tastes sweet under any name, sugar in those engineered forms is toxic to your body. [8.6, 8.7, 8.8]

Skewed perceptions of sweetness

Other related factors are the quantity of sweetness at which a certain food is perceived as sweet, as well as the source of that sweetness and any cultural meaning that may be attached to it (e.g., a special treat versus regular food). A ripe banana tastes sweeter than cooked brown rice; milk chocolate tastes sweeter than dark chocolate; ice cream tastes sweeter than cherries; maple syrup tastes sweeter than carrots. These can all be categorized as sweet-tasting foods, yet there is significant variation in the degree of their sweetness. Modern-day people often do not think of many fruits, vegetables, or brown rice as sweet foods. Their taste buds have become desensitized (usually by consuming too many sweets) to the point where something counts as sweet only if it contains added sugars – e.g., a cookie, but not a ripe fig – even though the latter may be sweeter by degree.

It is important therefore to choose foods that are either inherently sweet (lovingly supplied by Mother Nature) or sweetened with naturally derived sugars such as coconut sugar, honey, cane sugar, palm sugar, etc. Once you choose the *better alternative to artificially* (and chemically) sweetened foods and drinks, caution must also be exercised as to *how much* sugar you are consuming via that chosen food. Part of this is to observe the principle of *balancing natural sugars with fiber* – e.g., by eating the fruit itself, not merely drinking its juice – to avoid unknowingly overdosing on sugars (since an 8 oz. glass can hold the juice of several fruits!).

Ramifications of high sugar intake
The American Heart Association (AHA) has recommended *daily upper limits for added sugars*: for men – 9 tsp (38 g); for women – 6 tsp (25 g); for children above age 2 – 6 tsp (25 g); and for infants under 2 – zero grams. Some of these numbers may still be high by historical and evolutionary standards [8.9], not to mention that they do not take into account a person's individual constitution. However, a majority of people would still benefit if they *cut down* their sugar intake to such levels, as that would represent a solid improvement over an average person's daily sugar consumption in much of the world today.

To accomplish such a reduction, it would be wise to cultivate the habit of reading nutrition labels on food items (even if sweetened with naturally-derived sweeteners), to check how many grams of sugar are contained in one serving size of a particular food. You would be amazed that even innocuous-sounding foods (e.g., milk) often contain high doses of added sugars – mostly put there to appeal to desensitized taste buds and to compensate for the removal of other nutrients (e.g., in low-fat foods).

A host of serious health issues, including many chronic degenerative diseases, has been scientifically linked to the regular intake of foods that are high in *added sugars*. For example, sugar is the preferred food source that drives the growth of cancerous tumors, so cutting down on its consumption cuts off a cancer's supply line, and thus gives the body's immune system a better chance to properly recognize and remove the cancerous cells. [8.10] You will be pleasantly surprised to notice that if you regularly eat healthy, nutritious, and balanced meals, your desire for processed sweets will diminish greatly, thereby further reducing how much added sugars you consume (there is absolutely no need to reach the stated AHA limits), and thus helping to stabilize your health, to shed excess weight, and to once again properly sensitize your taste buds (so that they could become the reliable indicator that Nature intended for us). It may also be preferable to split sugar-containing foods across multiple meals, to avoid spiking your blood glucose levels.

Nature's candy store!
Wholesome, genuine forms of sweetness from natural foods such as carrots, yams, cooked beets, sweet onions, tomatoes, brown rice, cherries, blueberries, bananas, and grapes can greatly satisfy the inherent desire for a sweet taste. Adding such foods *consciously and regularly* to your diet will help to overcome cravings for unwholesome forms of sweet products, such as sodas, fruit juices, cereals, cookies, etc.

Even more sweetness into your life
A different, parallel form of wholesome, true sweetness can be experienced in nurturing, loving relationships. Humans are social creatures, and we all long for meaningful connections with others. If we are missing good company, this intense drive can often push us toward unhealthful forms of sweet foods as a replacement [8.11]. Then why not direct our energies instead toward cultivating loving relationships that in turn bring the natural sweetness back into our life experience, eliminating the need for "artificial sweetness"?

In conclusion, as we bring balance into our lives through consuming nutritious foods with a variety of different tastes, and enjoy a "sweet" relationship with ourselves and others, we can more reliably maintain optimum health for years to come.

~

One small action step you can take today: Replace your usual added-sugar treats with naturally sweet fruits and/or vegetables. Eat this way for three days. How is your energy level and mood? If you ate this way for three to four weeks, you will reprogram your taste buds, and your cravings for sugary foods will diminish. Are you willing to give it a try?

Need an added challenge? On a given day, every time you pick up a packaged food to eat, be it sweet or savory[13], read the nutrition label to check the amount of sugar contained in one serving size. Then on a piece of paper write the amount of sugar you just consumed based on how many servings you ate and/or drank. At the end of the day, tally the total amount of sugar you consumed. Continue doing this for a week. Did the results surprise you? If yes, how? If your sugar intake meets AHA's recommended daily limit, how could you further bring down your daily levels of added sugar?

---

[13] Note that savory foods can sometimes also contain some added sugars.

9: How do I find the right balance of raw versus cooked foods?

When it comes to achieving balance in any aspect of life, the principle of *moderation* (a.k.a. "the middle path") is a good guideline. This holds true when it comes to food choices. Let us look into the reasons for that: from an evolutionary perspective, as well as from a purely nutritional standpoint.

The evolutionary value of moderation

Over millennia, the human body slowly evolved to align with what humans needed to survive and what the environment was demanding and offering with respect to: nutrition, movement, activity, sleep, etc. For example, consider the life of eskimos. They eat much less fresh fruits and vegetables than the rest of us, and much more fatty animal proteins (from fish and seals). Their physical activity level is above that of people in most other cultures, and their sleep cycles (to adjust to the rhythms of day and night in the extreme north) are different, too. Their bodies have adapted to this regime over time. Their lifestyle is rooted in what their environment offers (in available food products, in daily hours of sunshine) and also what it demands (all due to the extremely cold temperatures).

Evolution is a *gradual process* that takes many generations to unfold. Therefore, we simply cannot afford to make a drastic (negative) change to any of these aspects within a single lifetime and yet expect good outcomes.

Consider these examples. Processed foods and foods containing artificial ingredients did not exist a few generations ago, so they are "unfamiliar" to a modern human's body systems. Consuming such foods, therefore, presents a major challenge to our digestive and elimination systems, "wearing" them out faster. Similarly, foods that contain high doses of sugar (especially added sugars, not naturally-grown fruits) are unnatural to our bodies too. Consuming extra sugar – as more and more people in our world have been doing lately, often unknowingly – over time overwhelms the pancreas and other essential organs, leading to conditions like insulin resistance and diabetes, among many other chronic degenerative diseases (virtually all rooted in processed sugar's inflammatory effect on a cellular level). [9.1, 9.2, 9.3]

To maintain good health, we must *abide by how human bodies have evolved* to function, and not depart in any significant ways. Otherwise we would introduce new stress factors and in the long run undercut our own health. As an analogy, you cannot fill up a gasoline car with diesel fuel, and expect it to run with the same efficiency and be highly functional for a long time. [9.4]

In large quantities, any (negative or even positive) aspect of food products and processes will understandably be *exaggerated*, thus presenting a potential health risk. In lower quantities, however, the body can handle challenges much better, cleansing itself more effectively, and sustaining less (or no) damage. Hence the value of regular detoxification processes (and fasting, as part of that [9.5]) – in order to give the body a break and allow a more complete internal cleansing to take place. However, such processes must be undertaken under competent supervision and care (to choose and monitor the right type of cleansing), since they too are uncommon to the modern human's body (i.e., most people do not know them well, nor practice them regularly).

Moderation in the choice of raw versus cooked foods
Our hunter-gatherer ancestors traditionally ate a mix of raw and cooked foods – including fruits, roots, meats, and so on. By necessity they ate with the seasons, as this was dictated by the availability of their food. We now understand some of the science behind why this was good for them and, respectively, beneficial for our own health today.

It starts with *awareness of the broader context* and *making regular informed adjustments*. Specifically, this means considering which food choices would:

(a) correspond to your own needs at a given time – based on your body type, age, activity, state of health, etc.;

(b) bring the right kind of energy to your body (e.g., calming, stimulating, creative, etc.);

(c) be appropriate for the geographical environment around you; and

(d) agree with the seasonal conditions around you; and so on.

All these aspects tend to dynamically change with time, suggesting the benefit of regularly revisiting your mix of selections.

Specifically, here is what each of the two categories brings:

Raw food benefits: Raw foods have a number of benefits in comparison to cooked foods:

- Raw foods generally retain more vitamins and anti-oxidants, since raw foods have not been subjected to a heating process that greatly diminishes those.

- Some (though not all) raw foods are easier to digest, since most of the necessary enzymes have been preserved (by not applying heat); otherwise the human digestive system would have to first reconstitute (i.e., recreate – which is taxing to the body) those enzymes in consumed food.

- Raw foods are closer to Nature, so throughout our evolution humans have become used to and accepting of many of them.

- Raw foods are closer to the state of being alive, and thus they can sustain another life (i.e., our lives) more readily.

- Raw foods can be sprouted, which converts them into a highly energetic, clean, and highly nutritive form.

- Raw foods can be fermented, rendering them easier to digest and helping to support healthy levels of good bacteria in the digestive tract.

- For raw foods that have not been mixed in with other ingredients, it may also be easier to recognize if any adulteration has happened (e.g., via additives, preservatives, colors, or other artificial ingredients).

Cooked food benefits: Cooked foods, in turn, have some benefits of their own compared to raw foods:

- The cooking process makes some (though not all) foods easier to digest, by softening the hard cell walls of vegetables like carrots, cabbage, etc.

- Cooking removes potentially harmful substances (e.g., goitrogens) from certain food items (e.g., potatoes, mushrooms, bean sprouts, celery, cruciferous vegetables – broccoli, Brussels sprouts, kale, etc.). [9.6]

- Cooking may offer an expanded set of food choices, especially for people who have meat and fish as part of their diets.

- Cooking dark green vegetables such as spinach, collard greens, kale, mustard greens, okra, asparagus, etc., helps to render nutrients such as iron and calcium more bio-available to your body.

- Whole grains and beans must be prepared properly by pre-soaking them before cooking, so as to remove harder to digest substances, such as lectins and phytates.

Once again, the key to robust health and wellbeing is in *moderation*, part of which is achieving a balance between types of foods we consume, including raw versus cooked. There is no magic number for what constitutes "balance" for you. To create your own balance, experiment with different proportions of raw and cooked foods to find out your personal equilibrium[14]. If your current diet is, for example, heavy on cooked foods, slowly introduce small amounts of raw foods, and increase over time while monitoring the effects and whether they are in alignment with your personal desired health / vitality goals.

～

---

[14] Even then, do not become attached to that "equilibrium" point, as it may change naturally over time, depending on the season, your activity level, and your own body's nourishment needs.

One small action step you can take today: Observe your typical eating habits for 3 days. Assess roughly and record daily what percentage of your food intake (meals and snacks) consists of raw foods and how much of it is cooked foods. Did the results surprise you? If yes, how? Are you satisfied with the way your eating habits are, or does it feel like your body is asking to make some changes? What *specific* steps do you feel guided to take?

Need an added challenge? For one day, commit to eating only raw foods for all your meals and snacks. (Doing this may require some planning.) Observe how you feel at the end of the day and on the next morning. Do you notice any difference in your energy levels, mood, cravings, and sleep pattern? The very next day, commit to eating only (healthy) cooked foods for all your meals and snacks. Once again, observe how you feel at the end of that day and on the morning after that. How different are your energy levels, mood, cravings, and sleep pattern? What did you learn about yourself through this exercise? Where is your personal equilibrium now?

10: I eat vegetarian / vegan food as a conscious choice. Are there valid concerns I need to be aware of and plan for?

The vegetarian argument revisited

Some people choose a vegetarian or vegan diet[15] due to ethical concerns with animal-based diets, e.g., the inhumane treatment of animals in concentrated and confined industrial operations (CAFOs) and the environmentally unsustainable operation of the meat-based industry. Others make that choice for its perceived health benefits – plant foods generally contain high levels of anti-oxidants, minerals, and fiber, while animal-based foods often contain concentrated toxins[16]. [10.1]

There is yet another important, less well known, argument in favor of vegetarian (and vegan) diets. As you already know, *you become what you eat.* The foods you consume literally become *building blocks* for your cells, tissues, organs, blood, etc. When you eat a predominantly plant-based diet, its building blocks can be re-integrated (re-imprinted) more effectively and efficiently (compared to animal-derived foods) into your human body, because the plant kingdom is farther away on the *evolutionary level of consciousness* from Homo Sapiens (human species). In contrast, mammals and other animals are much closer (i.e., more similar) to humans in their evolutionary level of consciousness, so the animal proteins you absorb when ingesting meats are harder to properly re-imprint as your own (i.e., to become part of your body). This means that the digestive and absorption processes for animal-based foods will be much more taxing on the human body and also much less effective – you will be taking on the cellular memory of another (animal) being that became your food. [10.2]

---

[15] Generally, the term "vegetarian" is used to refer to a person (or diet) that avoids meat and fish, while "vegan" refers to a person (or diet) that in addition to that also avoids any animal-based products, including dairy, eggs, etc.

[16] Toxins concentrate especially in the flesh of animals that are higher on the food chain. Toxins also accumulate due to the stress effects on animals held in confinement, as well as during the slaughtering process.

Finally, research indicates that people with certain body constitutions (e.g., blood type, activity level, etc.) may need an animal-based diet during at least parts of their lives (e.g., due to regular high physical activity, due to living in regions with cold weather, etc.) in order to function. It is important, therefore, to *not be dogmatic* in making the choice, but to consider what really serves you (and any children around you) best in your particular environment and life context.

Key nutrients and minerals

Regardless of dietary preferences (vegetarian, meat-eater, or any other), you must still *pay conscious and close attention* to the foods you select daily. For optimum health, it is important to take in foods that collectively give your body *all the essential nutrients and minerals*, in order to maintain proper balance.

For people who choose to be vegetarians and vegans, this consideration matters too, because key nutrients and minerals such as calcium, iodine, iron, and vitamin B_{12} – all of which your body needs to thrive – are more sparsely found throughout the plant kingdom. For your body to obtain these in good balance, you need to eat a wide variety of plant-based and vegetarian sources (e.g., vegetables and fruits of many colors; sea vegetables and seaweeds; legumes; some whole grains; and fats / oils from olives, coconuts, avocados, ghee, or butter[17]). For vegans especially, it may be best to supplement some of these minerals (e.g., vitamin B_{12}), since scientists claim that they do not naturally occur in sufficient quantities in plants. For other minerals on the above list, there are adequate plant-based sources, as listed in the following chart:

Mineral	Plant-based sources
iodine (I)	sea vegetables and seaweeds (kelp, kombu, dulse, etc.), Himalayan crystal salt, dried prunes, cranberries, navy beans, plain yogurt, etc.

---

[17] You may see other authors add palm fruit oil to this list. While palm fruit oil (not palm kernel oil, which does not digest well) is considered a "superfood," its production is ecologically unsustainable, displacing tropical rainforests, and thus causing harm on a global scale. Given so many other good options, we do not recommend palm fruit oil.

Mineral	Plant-based sources
iron (Fe)	dates, raisins, lentils, peas, brown rice, quinoa, Brussels sprouts, (cooked) spinach, spirulina, tempeh, pumpkin seeds, etc.
calcium (Ca)	broccoli, kale, fennel, blackstrap molasses, tempeh, amaranth, turnip greens, sesame, almonds, quinoa, chickpeas, prunes, etc.

Finally, *do not be a "vegetarian junkie."* Take care to select only the highest quality vegetarian / vegan foods, and ensure variety. Even French fries, soda, and sweetened breakfast cereals technically constitute vegetarian choices, but they are not nearly as nutritious and indeed are quite far from being healthy choices. Similarly, a consistently limited selection of vegetables, fruits, and grains – as in the modern diet of many people in East Asian countries, for example – would be an unhealthy diet, even though it is otherwise vegetarian. The resulting deficiency of essential macro- and micronutrients in such a diet (except for carbohydrates, from rice as a staple food) would lead to long-term imbalances, often with lifelong adverse consequences, especially for young children.

It should be noted that none of this is hard to do right. The need for extra care is not an argument against vegetarian or vegan diets. It simply requires proper planning and preparation on your part.

Extra caution for children's diets

Children's bodies and brains develop intensively, so a *steady supply* of key nutrients is needed for proper growth. Hence, caution must be exercised when a child chooses – due to ethical reasons, peer pressure, or perceived health benefits – a diet, including meat-based, vegetarian, or vegan.

Drastic dietary changes or restrictions are generally not recommended for anyone (except under the careful supervision of a licensed health care practitioner), and especially not for children. When a change in the diet feels desirable (e.g., toward, or away from, vegetarian / vegan), remember that "one size does not fit all" and dogmatic approaches tend to be unproductive – including when it comes to nutrition. Take a *personalized approach* instead, considering aspects like one's blood type, age, gender, activity level, long-term habits, access to a variety of plant-based foods, etc. Use the flexible "trial and error" approach – choosing (or helping a child to choose) to follow a new (e.g., vegetarian) diet for a certain period of time (e.g., 2-4 weeks[18]) while carefully observing the experiences. The feedback from this can be your guide as to whether, and to what extent, the new diet serves you and/or your child well.

~

One small action step you can take today: Pick a day this week to go fully vegetarian or vegan ("Meatless Mondays" or "Sattvic Saturdays," perhaps?). Notice how you feel in your body, mind, and spirit at the end of that day. Did you notice any shifts? Was this an easy exercise for you? Why or why not? Would you consider eating a vegetarian diet, at least one day a week? What healthy vegetarian alternatives would you pick?

Need an added challenge? For an entire week, eat a strictly vegetarian or vegan diet and also eliminate all processed forms of vegetarian foods such as chips, breakfast cereals, French fries, etc. How do you feel at the end of that week – physically, mentally, and emotionally? Are you experiencing any unusual cravings, or perhaps are you having less of the cravings you had before? Do you believe that your plate is balanced – including all the major food groups that are in alignment with your body's constitution? What small change can you make to your vegetarian / vegan diet in order to give you even more nourishment?

---

[18] To really see results of your changes, you generally need more than a few days.

11: Is eating meat healthy or harmful for my body? I hear conflicting messages – that eating meat is bad for me, but that I "must" eat meat to get adequate protein. Where is the truth?

In its basic meaning, the term "meat" refers to animal flesh, primarily that of mammals.[19] Many people in Western countries associate meat with beef, while referring to other forms of animal flesh as pork (for pigs), poultry (for chickens, turkeys, ducks), venison (for deer), escargot (for snails), etc. For the purposes of answering this question more completely, we choose to use the term "meat" to mean animal flesh, in general.

Animal-based versus plant-based proteins

Meats are particularly popular as a food because they are sources of protein, which are primary building blocks of the human body, forming your cells, organs, muscles, tendons, hair, etc. Proteins are made of smaller units called amino acids, which are attached to one another in long chains. 22 different types of amino acids have been identified, and they link together in numerous combinations to make functional[20] proteins. The human body can synthesize 13 of these amino acids, whereas the remaining 9 need to be obtained exclusively from food sources (hence they are called essential amino acids). Foods containing all 9 essential amino acids are called "complete proteins." Most of the known complete proteins are obtained from food sources such as fish, eggs, meat, poultry, and dairy.

Plant-based proteins are generally considered "incomplete," because many (but not all) of them lack one or more essential amino acids. Still, there exist many plant-based sources of complete proteins – only the quantities of each essential amino acid in them may not be sufficient to deliver the amount of complete protein needed for the daily nutrition of humans. Examples of plant foods that have at least

---

[19] Some people colloquially use the word "meat" to also refer to the edible parts of fruits and nuts. This secondary meaning of the word is not the authors' intent in this book.

[20] A functional protein refers to a protein that supports structural, mechanical, and metabolic processes.

some of the essential amino acids are: quinoa (a complete protein itself), kidney beans, chickpeas (a.k.a. garbanzo beans), black beans[21], pumpkin seeds, cashews, pistachios, soy beans[22], black-eyed peas, cauliflower, spirulina, potatoes, and so on. Incomplete proteins must be eaten in combination with other foods in order to become complete (e.g., rice and beans form a complete protein when eaten together, within the same day). In general, grains combined with nuts, seeds, or beans can deliver complete proteins. [11.2, 11.3]

When is eating meat unhealthy for you?
There are several influencing factors, most of which are also closely interrelated.

The modern face of animal farming
Animal farming has drastically changed from the days of our ancestors, with the advent of modern industrial agriculture. In earlier times, meat was acquired quite differently, ranging from hunting in the wild (by early man) for basic survival, to raising animals in local farms (by modern man) where the animals grazed in open lands and were well cared for until they were deemed ready for slaughter. However, since the 1970s animals have increasingly been bred and raised in unnatural settings. Animal farming has been made to resemble a factory; hence the term "factory farming" to describe this method of raising animals for human consumption. In the factory farming method (a.k.a. concentrated animal feeding operations – CAFOs), hundreds of animals are permanently confined to very small spaces and are given feed that is not their natural diet (e.g., grain for cattle, instead of grass or hay) and has also become genetically modified (e.g., corn, alfalfa) lately. Animals are administered artificial growth hormones to make them grow to sizes they would naturally not grow to, and in relatively short durations as well. They are also regularly given antibiotics,

---

[21] Note that black beans, as commonly prepared in the Western world today, are high in glutamate, a harmful compound in large quantities, driving the growth of cancer cells. [11.1]

[22] To avoid causing harm, soy must be non-GMO, and also prepared via fermentation or sprouting. Many soy-based products sold in the West today do not meet these criteria. Additionally, soy is relatively harder to digest, so it may not be a good option for people with a compromised digestive ability.

partly to fend off adverse reactions to the unnatural diet as well as any potential contamination. Due to all these practices, a much larger number of artificially "fattened" animals are ready for the "market" in a short span of time. The intent is to reduce a factory farm's time-to-market, and hence to increase the CAFO's profitability.

Infected meat and large scale use of antibiotics
Such CAFOs (factory farms) are often a *breeding ground for infection due to contamination*. Due to the confined spaces and the associated stress, animals tend to peck or dig their horns into each other, thereby hurting one another and leading to infections. Infection in one animal can easily spread across many more due to their sheer number and proximity, and may contaminate large batches of meat during processing. Antibiotics are therefore routinely added to the feed, partly to reduce the chance of bacterial infections. The resulting antibiotic-laden manure is often used as fertilizer, which spreads contamination to wider areas. [11.4]

Meat becomes imprinted in you
As you consume meat from factory farms, there is not only the inherent danger of taking in contaminated meat (e.g., from Salmonella, E-coli), but also the hormones and antibiotics administered to these animals will end up in your body and over time become the building blocks for your cells, organs, muscles, etc. Additionally, the ill treatment of animals in confinement creates chronic fear and panic in animals, triggering their own fight-or-flight hormones, which then get transferred to you when you eat their meat. As you can imagine, such meat has lower nutritive value. [11.5, 11.6] *You really become a product of what (meat) you eat*, at all levels – physical, mental, emotional, and spiritual.

For completeness, let us state that dairy products and eggs from CAFOs, as well as conventionally farmed fish, are similarly affected – and will negatively affect you, in turn, if you consume such products.

Natural resources become polluted and depleted
A number of industrial agriculture processes hurt the delicate ecological balance and biodiversity. Fertilizer runoff, fecal matter, and urine from CAFO animals drain into waterways and pollute them. Rainforests, the "lungs" of planet Earth, are cleared over time

to make room for expanding factory farms. Toxic mercury from industries, hospitals, power plants, and other sources ends up in the flesh of fish[23] that you may later consume, thus adversely impacting not only water bodies and aquatic life, but also directly your health.

Oversized portions of meat

Many people these days consume *large portions of meat at every meal*[24] and hence get much more protein than their bodies need for optimal functioning. This further adds up if you include eggs and dairy as other common protein sources. Excess protein consumption on a regular basis, however, has been linked to certain types of cancer. According to The National Health and Nutrition Examination Survey [11.7], Americans consume almost twice the daily-recommended intake established by the Food and Nutrition Board. The suggested daily intake of protein for an adult is 0.36 g of protein per pound of body weight (e.g., if you weigh 150 pounds, your RDA (recommended daily allowance) of protein will be 54 g per day). For children, it is suggested that they consume 0.5 g of protein per pound of body weight (e.g., if a child weighs 60 pounds, his/her RDA of protein will be 30 g per day). [11.8, 11.9] Note, however, that *protein is not the same as meat*, so at least some of the above recommended daily allowances for protein must come from other sources. Centenarian cultures have been limiting their animal protein intake to 10%. [11.2]

Not all meats are created equal

Meats from CAFO-raised animals are best avoided. In addition, some animals' flesh is a particularly dirty source[25] of meat (e.g., pork; fish without scales: catfish, eel, etc.), even if raised sustainably.

When does eating meat become less problematic for you?

Here are some considerations, if you choose to consume meat regularly:

---

[23] Fish that is higher in the food chain, mostly larger fish (e.g., tuna, swordfish, sea bass, etc.), have higher mercury contamination of the flesh, so it is best avoided or minimized.

[24] What if, instead, people considered meat as simply "garnish," supplementing other protein choices, not dominating?

[25] It clogs up vital energy channels (chakras) in the human body. [11.10]

- Farms and ranches exist where animals are treated more humanely. They are allowed to graze or move about freely in open pastures, and to eat foods according to their natural instincts (i.e., cattle eating grass, chicken eating barley and corn, etc.). Meat from such *pasture-raised and/or organically or grass-fed animals that are well cared for* is higher in nutritive value (e.g., higher omega-3 fatty acids, beta-carotene, vitamin E, CLA – conjugated linoleic acid, etc.), and the quality of that meat (e.g., free of hormones and antibiotics) is superior to that of its factory farmed counterpart. [11.5]

- Take into consideration your individual constitution and life situation. For example, your protein needs will be greater if you are a nursing mother or a convalescent, while such needs will be respectively lower if you lead a sedentary lifestyle or are among the elderly. However, please note again that *protein does not equal meat*: unlike some of your hunter-gatherer ancestors for whom meat was a necessity for survival, you do have other protein options. *Do not exceed your recommended daily allowance* when deciding how much meat you consume.

- If you are an *"O" blood type*, your body has much better digestive strength (provided it is not compromised due to poor eating habits such as by consuming highly processed and junk foods) than the other blood types. Specifically, this helps to more efficiently metabolize the cholesterol, proteins, and fats contained in animal products. This trait for "O" blood types is primarily due to: (a) a tendency towards having higher levels of stomach acid; and (b) higher levels of two key chemicals in the body – intestinal alkaline phosphatase enzyme and ApoB48 lipoprotein. These two factors not only help "O" blood types digest meat better, but also increase their ability to heal their digestive tract and to better assimilate calcium. [11.11]

Even if you consume meat only from organic, grass-fed animals, pasture-raised in local, small farms:

- the fear and panic hormones of animals around the time of slaughter are still ingested by you;

- meat is still harder for your body to re-imprint as your own proteins, as animals are much closer to humans in their evolutionary level of consciousness (this is discussed in more detail in §10).

- you may feel heavier and more sluggish after a meat-containing meal (because meat takes longer than plant-based food to be processed by the human digestive system), making the meal less effective than available wholesome protein alternatives[26], especially if you wish to engage in a variety of dynamic physical activities. However, if you are an "O" blood type and/or consume meats sparingly, both in quantity and frequency, this may mitigate the issue of heaviness.

- the natural resources used to produce a pound of meat are still much greater than those required for the production of other (nutritionally comparable) protein sources – making it unsustainable ecologically as a food source for large human populations. [11.12]

- you still need to consume it very sparingly, and to account for the total quantity of all protein sources you consume daily.

- the quantity of meat you ingest makes the difference between nourishment and poison.

In a nutshell

To achieve and maintain good health, *include a variety of protein sources* in your diet, and among them some plant-based protein-rich foods. There exist much better options (for you and for the environment) than meats from industrially-raised (CAFO) animals, plus any meat production requires large areas of land as grazing grounds for cattle or for chickens to roam freely. Additionally, many more natural resources overall are used up to produce a pound of meat, compared to a pound of another protein source. Therefore, a meat-based diet is unsustainable ecologically, especially if a large human population consumes predominantly that.

---

[26] Avoid highly processed, textured, "meatless" meats, e.g., tofurky, soy-based chorizo, etc.

~

One small action step you can take today: Calculate your recommended daily protein limit (from the formula given above), and eat only up to that amount of protein each day for three days. Take into account the various sources from which you plan on getting your protein. You would be surprised how quickly they all add up to your recommended daily limit! What did you learn from this exercise? How did you feel, overall? Were you faced with some interesting revelations? If yes, what were they?

Need an added challenge? For one week, have your meals alternate between good quality animal protein and complete protein from vegetarian sources, e.g., animal protein for breakfast, vegetarian protein for lunch, etc. Please include vegetables and good fats as part of this balanced plate of food. Here again, do not exceed your recommended daily protein intake. How differently do you feel when you eat animal proteins versus plant proteins? Would you consider expanding the variety of sources of protein in your diet? If yes, what would be your choices?

12: Lately, I see that a lot of people prefer to go gluten-free. Is gluten bad for me?

Gluten is the name of a protein found in all varieties (durum, emmer, spelt, kamut, einkorn, etc.) and forms (semolina, farro, etc.) of wheat, and also in barley, rye, and triticale (a hybrid of wheat and rye). The word "gluten" comes from Latin, and refers to gluten's glue-like properties, which make it easier to fashion products out of the grains. Of all gluten-containing grains, wheat is the most popular and most widely grown on Earth. In total, wheat takes up more acreage on the planet than any other crop. [12.1]

The modern kind(s) of wheat
The wheat grain has undergone massive changes since ancient times. The earliest known cultivated wheat (called einkorn) is considered relatively easier to digest than most modern varieties, since its DNA is a diploid species – with two sets of chromosomes (i.e., a simpler structure), similar to a human's diploid chromosomal structure. About 2000 years later, in order to increase the yield of gluten per harvest (and thus produce more units of any wheat product due to the higher density of gluten), emmer was created by hybridization, resulting in a wheat variety that has four sets of chromosomes, making it tetraploid. Spelt was later introduced through further hybridization, and it contains six sets of chromosomes, making it hexaploid. Today, there are complex wheat varieties with up to 32 (or perhaps more!) sets of chromosomes. [12.2, 12.3]

As hybridizations continued over the millennia, the gluten content went up significantly in each successive wheat variety, thereby introducing many more (and many kinds of) proteins in the wheat. Due to such an explosive increase in the gluten proteins, today's wheat is no longer as easily broken down in the human gut, as it is not (yet) recognized by the human genome. This may be contributing to health issues such as celiac disease and non-celiac gluten sensitivity, in addition to triggering other chronic illnesses including diabetes, heart disease, and arthritis, among others. The gut's inability to break down complex proteins is a condition that is further exacerbated by several factors: the parallel increase in the modern consumption of processed foods; the presence of more pollutants and chemical toxicities in our bodies; and other self-made (ecological, technological, hormonal, etc.) imbalances that wreak havoc on our digestive systems.

The modern processing of wheat

In addition to the rampant hybridization of seeds, the method of processing wheat into finished products (such as bread, pasta, etc.) has also undergone tremendous changes since the times of our ancestors. For example, sourdough bread used to take two days to prepare properly; today, a form of sourdough bread is often ready in two hours due to shortening of the natural fermentation process via the addition of starters, cultures, and other "unnatural" elements, all intended to yield a finished product (and the associated profit) in less and less time.

In ancient cultures, grains were commonly prepared in ways that deactivated or reduced any anti-nutrients, thereby allowing humans to receive the grain's full nutritional benefit, while also rendering grain products easier on the digestive system. The two anti-nutrients present in grains are phytates (acids) and lectins (proteins). Phytates are compounds that bind up minerals, and this prevents full mineral absorption by the body when grains are ingested. Lectins are a type of protein that binds to cell membranes (insulin receptors), and since they are not digestible our immune systems produce antibodies against them. Phytates can be deactivated, wholly or partially, and the lectin content can be reduced through soaking, sprouting, or souring (a.k.a. fermenting) the grains, which in turn increases the bioavailability of key minerals such as magnesium, calcium, zinc, iron, etc., and also makes the resulting grains easier to digest for the human system. [12.4, 12.5]

Such careful measures for preparing grains used to be implemented by ancient cultures, but the process has since changed drastically. With the advent of industrialized agriculture came progressive loss and neglect of such ancient wisdom. Many food manufacturers, chefs, and even home cooks do not take the time to prepare grains (and other related products such as bread) properly, which makes the result nutritionally deficient and harder to digest. Adding to this compromised way of processing, many modern flours undergo a "refinement" process in which the bran and germ that contain key nutrients are removed. Flours also often go through a bleaching process, using a chlorine gas bath (with chlorine oxide) for the purposes of whitening (i.e., for cosmetic reasons). Then, instead of allowing the flour to normally age with time, it is quickly "aged" to improve the gluten (binding together) and baking quality. [12.6] All these techniques for processing whole wheat grains further add to the burden placed on our (already partially compromised) digestion.

Although corn and rice are technically also known to contain some gluten, the primary difference is that the gluten in them is water soluble, unlike in wheat, barley, rye, and triticale where it is not. Grains containing water soluble gluten break down in water and hence are relatively easier to digest.

Gluten deconstructed

Gluten contains two proteins – glutenin and gliadin. The one that people predominantly have a negative reaction to is gliadin. Gliadin is known to create an opiate-like effect in the body, abnormally stimulating the appetite and inducing cravings for low-quality (junk) carbohydrates like cakes, cookies, etc., instead of healthier alternatives. If you regularly succumb to such cravings, your body will experience high blood sugar and high blood insulin levels, over time leading to chronic diseases such as diabetes. Gliadin is also known to cause inflammation and increase bowel permeability, thereby causing leaky gut syndrome and other digestive disorders. [12.7] Wheat germ agglutinin (WGA) is the lectin of wheat that causes intestinal toxicity. [12.8] It behaves like super glue: it binds to everything and also prevents the metabolism of vitamin D, itself an essential ingredient for boosting the immune system and preventing chronic diseases such as cancer. WGA can get into the cells of your body and can also cross the protective blood-brain barrier, thereby leading to neurological disorders as well, including dementia, ataxia, neuropathy, myopathy, etc. [12.9]

Is gluten a problem for every person?

The answer, as is the case for many questions of a general nature, is not clearly black or white. One needs to consider the presence of: (a) apparent and easily recognizable symptoms / reactions; (b) subtle(r) and mild(er) reactions; and (c) indirect symptoms / reactions of ingesting gluten. Let us look at each of these three broad categories:

(a) *Apparent and easily recognizable symptoms / reactions* – If you experience any moderate to severe symptoms or reactions, either immediately or within 24 hours of ingesting or coming in contact with gluten, then it is highly likely that you are having an allergic response to the respective food. One of the predominant allergic responses people may have to the ingestion of (or any form of contact with) gluten is Celiac disease. In this condition, the immune system attacks both the gluten proteins and the body's own intestinal walls, hence it is classified as an autoimmune disease. The symptoms may be of varying degrees and types: e.g., digestive issues such as bloating, stomach pain, diarrhea, etc.; fatigue; bone and joint pain; anxiety; failure to thrive; anemia; nutritional deficiencies due to the degeneration of the intestinal walls; and more. The incidence of Celiac disease has quadrupled in the last 40-50 years, which could be due to the changes in gliadin's genetic sequence over the years due to the hybridization of wheat. (Certain genetic sequences were absent in the wheat strains of the 1950's and 1960's, but are present in almost all modern wheat strains.)

(b) *Subtle(r) and mild(er) symptoms / reactions* – If you experience any mild to moderate symptoms or reactions between 24 and 72 hours after ingesting or coming in contact with gluten, then it is likely that you have a sensitivity or intolerance to gluten. Some of the symptoms of non-Celiac gluten sensitivity are quite similar to those for Celiac disease (e.g., bloating, diarrhea, stomach pain, bone and joint aches and pains, etc.); others include skin disorders such as eczema, brain fog, moodiness, among others.

(c) *Indirect symptoms / reactions* – If you experience virtually no palpable symptoms or reactions after ingesting or coming in contact with gluten, then there is a chance that gluten may be agreeable to your body. However, many people who are apparently allergy-free and can tolerate gluten tend to over time develop symptoms indicative of the onset of some chronic disease (e.g., diabetes, heart disease, arthritis, thyroiditis, digestive disorders, or other types of inflammation). Such health conditions may be related to the regular ingestion of gluten over a period of time.

If you suspect that you have some of the above symptoms / reactions, consider eliminating the suspect – wheat and other forms of gluten-containing grains – for up to 6 weeks and then reintroduce gluten at the end of that elimination period, to observe if there is reappearance of the symptoms / reactions. This is one of the best tests to truly ascertain if gluten is problematic for you or not. There are other sophisticated tests as well (such as those offered by Cyrex Laboratories – www.cyrexlabs.com). Specific blood tests also exist to check for IgE (immunoglobulin E) antibodies – those get activated if the body experiences any food intolerances. In blood tests, however, there is a significant chance for false negatives (and false positives, too) in the results, making it hard to draw definitive correct conclusions. The above mentioned *elimination diet* is by far the most non-invasive, yet trusted, method for checking if you have allergies / sensitivities to gluten and/or other allergenic foods.

Should you stop eating wheat products?
Much research exists (as quoted above) that evidences the harm to the human body from consuming wheat and other gluten-containing grains. However, less well understood is the fact that a truly healthy organism has a *well-tuned internal environment*, conducive to digesting and assimilating even such grains.

If you commit to creating a strong internal environment within yourself, you may be able to still eat good quality wheat and other glutinous grains, *in moderation*. In that case, you will be best served to choose grains that are non-hybridized, organically grown, unbleached, and properly prepared by soaking, sprouting, or souring (fermenting).

Also important is that wheat and most gluten-containing grains withstand cold temperatures well, so historically they have been preserved as food for the winter months (after harvesting in the fall), when other types of foods are less available. Humans' digestive fire (i.e., digestive enzymes in the saliva and gut, hydrochloric acid in the stomach, etc.) has also evolved over the ages to be stronger in the colder months, enabling proper break-down of harder-to-digest glutens. Hence, consuming gluten *seasonally* (and not throughout the year, as we are used to in modern times) is another way to improve your health outcomes with wheat and other gluten-containing grains.

Maintaining a healthy internal environment is crucial
In the end, if you wish to enjoy vibrant health and wellbeing, then creating an optimal internal environment is a necessary first step before introducing foods known to be difficult to digest.

The health of your internal environment is primarily determined by the health of your digestive system, including your gut health and intestinal microbiome (i.e., the presence of beneficial bacteria). To a large extent, maintaining good health internally is under your control. Your external environment, in contrast, contains many harmful substances that are largely out of your direct control. This includes: chemicals (in food and non-food products), pollutants (in the air, soil, water, etc.), genetically engineered foods (and the pesticides they are grown with), prescription medications (which have been observed to leach in public water supply systems), antibiotics (which hurt humans' good intestinal flora along with their targets), etc. All these can combine to seriously and adversely upset the equilibrium of your internal environment. [12.10] Your appropriate choices of food, water, and lifestyle behaviors can help you to minimize the negative effect of the external factors.

The cleaner and more consciously you live, the lesser any negative influences on your health would be from your food and non-food choices. Detoxing / cleansing regularly (at least twice a year) is one way to remove built-up toxins from your physical body, as well as from your emotional and mental bodies; as a result you "make room" for healthy foods, emotions, and thoughts to be naturally and easily assimilable by your system. Simple detoxes and cleanses can be easily done at home: e.g., intermittent fasts, elimination diets, juicing, etc. For more intense detoxes / cleanses, however, please consult an expert or your health care provider before embarking on those, to ensure that your results are as positive as you intend them to be.

Gluten-free options
If you choose to (or are advised to) reduce or avoid consumption of gluten, know that several wholesome and nutritious gluten-free grain options are available. Among them are: quinoa, buckwheat, rice (e.g., brown, basmati, jasmine), millet, amaranth, sorghum, teff, gluten-free

oats, and others. Even so, some gluten-free options are not as healthful due to one or more of the following reasons:

- high glycemic index – due to heavy processing (e.g., in potato, corn, tapioca, and arrowroot starches) and/or added sugars (e.g., to avoid a taste "like cardboard");

- GMO – e.g., soy and corn are popular gluten-free substitutes, but if their source is not organic, they are likely genetically modified;

- thickeners and/or gums – highly processed ingredients, commonly added to recreate the glue-like properties of the missing gluten (e.g., in xanthan gum, gellan gum); and

- cross-contamination from gluten-containing grains – if not explicitly stated on the label as being "certified gluten-free."

In the event that you accidently consume gluten-containing ingredients, there are interventions available to you as a "first aid." [12.11] Check out the referenced link for details.

Trust your body awareness
It will serve you well to remind yourself time and again that it is vital to pay attention to how your body feels (a.k.a., body awareness) – when you eat certain foods or when you stop eating certain foods – rather than blindly following fads. The gluten-free product industry is a $16 billion industry, growing rapidly. [12.12] As such, they have a vested interest in having people believe that their products are superior in most or all situations.

Your body may, however, be different in special ways. There are no "right" or "wrong" foods to eat, especially if you have taken the time to source foods that are whole, organic, and minimally processed, and if your digestive system is in good health. Observe how *your* unique body processes such (whole and organic, whether gluten-free or not) foods, when consumed regularly. If you find that you need to make any adjustments to re-balance your body, boldly take the necessary steps in that direction.

Gluten beyond foods

Owing to its glue-like properties, gluten is also widely used as an industrial adhesive, as well as in many personal care products (e.g., shampoo, make-up, lotion, toothpaste, etc.), medicines, supplements, pet foods, etc. So if you opt to go gluten-free, pay close attention to gluten's potential presence in not only food ingredients, but also in other products that you regularly use. [12.13]

~

One small action step you can take today: For one day experiment with products made from gluten-free whole grains. Choose ones you have never tried before. Some options are: quinoa, buckwheat, amaranth, sorghum, millet, and brown rice. Prepare them according to a recipe you like (easy-to-prepare breakfast options exist, too). Did you like your gluten-free meals? Which grain was your favorite, and why? Would you be open to adding such new ingredients into your regular diet? Which of your favorite gluten-containing recipes are you open to re-creating using gluten-free grains?

Need an added challenge? Try one or more methods – soaking, sprouting, or fermenting – of preparing gluten-containing grains in their whole, unrefined version. If you are on a strictly gluten-free diet, then choose to do the same for the whole grain version of any gluten-free grain of your choice. Which method(s) of preparation did you choose? How differently did your food taste compared to your usual way of preparing it? Was your serving size bigger or smaller than usual? Why do you think this was so? What did you feel immediately after, and then a few days after, eating the grains prepared in your chosen method(s)? How do you feel about eating such minimally processed and traditionally prepared whole grains?

13: Today I see so many non-dairy options. Do I need to be concerned about cow's milk?

Our traditional agrarian lifestyle

After following a hunter-gatherer way of life for two million years, human cultures began to settle down and start domesticating plants and animals about 12,500 years ago. This marked the beginning of the agricultural revolution. People had access to milk from domesticated animals, and to grains from their farmlands. The animals also helped our ancestors in farming work: ploughing, towing, etc. Therefore ancient cultures had great reverence for their domesticated animals. Milk from these animals was the primary source of dietary protein. People had easy access to the purest, highly nutritive, unprocessed form of milk, as the animals grazed in open pastures and were well cared for by their "owners." [13.1]

Advent of the dairy "industry" and related processes

The advent of the industrial revolution in the mid-18th century led to replacing more and more open farmlands with factories, and the human (and animal) workforce – with machines. [13.2] These changes gave birth to new manufacturing and production processes, thereby launching what we now call the "factory setting." The face of agriculture changed, and with it also the dairy farming, lately known as the "dairy industry."

In a factory setting with machinery and mechanical processes taking over milking, storage, distribution, etc., preserving the freshness of milk became an important consideration. In contrast to early agrarian times, 18th century consumers lived in locations farther away from where the milk was produced. Hence, the technique of pasteurization[27] of dairy was invented, in order to increase its shelf life under refrigeration by slowing or preventing the growth of microorganisms that spoil the milk. It was Louis Pasteur who in the late 1800s invented pasteurization in connection with his studies on germ theory of diseases. Following his research, a regulation for

---

[27] In the pasteurization process, milk is heated to 162F for 15 seconds, thereby destroying harmful microorganisms (mostly bacteria). Thus treated, milk generally stays fresh under refrigeration for about 3-4 weeks.

mandatory milk pasteurization was passed by the U.S. government in 1920. [13.3]

Engineering an increased demand for dairy products

In today's culture, the consumption of dairy (especially cow's milk) products such as milk, cheese, and yogurt has increased significantly. Milk is considered by many to be a rich source of calcium, necessary for optimum bone health and for preventing osteoporosis. Various food pyramids created by USDA over the course of several decades have all suggested that a person needs up to 3 servings of milk (i.e., 3 regular cups of 8 oz.) each day. [13.4] Dairy corporations and farmers with a vested interest (i.e., more milk sales means larger profits to them) in the industrialization of dairy farming have been exercising significant influence over governments in designing policies and recommendations, including placing dairy products in a prominent position on the food pyramids. Through shrewd marketing strategies (e.g., slogans such as "Milk your diet" and "Got milk?") and with the implied health benefits of milk, people have been encouraged to consume ever larger quantities of milk products daily. This has aided the push toward selling more and more dairy, including in its highly processed forms (e.g., ice creams, puddings, shakes, smoothies, creamy coffee drinks, etc.).

Enticing kids with fancy dairy products

To further increase the sales of milk products, dairy companies have sought to appeal more to kids, who are often the most gullible and vulnerable. Moreover, habituating ("brainwashing") kids from a young age is a strategy to ensure they stay on as customers well into their adulthood too. Many different flavors of milk and yogurt have sprung up, often containing artificial colors, flavors, and added refined sugars. Such highly sweetened (with up to 23 grams of sugar per serving!) and flavored milk and yogurt has in some places even become an accepted part of a so called "healthy" school lunch. From the previous discussion on sugary foods in §8, you are well aware of the negative ramifications of consuming large quantities of added sugars, not to mention the added artificial colors and flavors that further exacerbate this problem.

Unnatural methods of milk production and their effects

To sell more and more dairy, corporations have needed a steady supply of large quantities of milk year-round. But how could they manage to produce so much milk from cows that naturally give milk only when they bear calves and even then for a limited time only? Two primary methods have been employed to achieve the high milk production goals (on average, 9 gallons per day from each cow). Both methods are unnatural and have significant negative ramifications:

(a) *Artificial insemination* – Cows are impregnated through artificial insemination while they are still lactating from their previous pregnancy. This enables a corporation to milk such cows for about 10 months per year.

However, the milk from cows that are two months pregnant contains 5 times more estrogen than milk from non-pregnant cows. Cows closer to full-term pregnancy have 33 times the levels of estrogen of their non-pregnant counterparts. Regularly consuming milk that contains such high levels of sex hormones, such as estrogen, has been shown to have negative effects on human health – increasing the incidence of prostate, uterine, and ovarian cancers; mammary tumors; lowering testosterone levels; and affecting the sexual maturation of pre-pubertal children. [13.5]

(b) *Administering bovine growth hormone (rBGH / rBST)* – A genetically engineered growth hormone is injected into cows every week, to force them to produce larger quantities of milk than what their bodies are naturally designed to produce. Because rBGH or rBST is similar to a hormone that cows naturally produce in their bodies, regularly boosting the levels of this mimicking artificial hormone has the effect of increasing cows' milk production many-fold.

Forcing cows to produce more milk than what Nature intended for them may cause mastitis, an udder infection that can increase pus formation and its accumulation in the milk. Pus cell counts have been shown to average up to 332 million per glass of milk – well above what humans can safely take in. This may lead to conditions such as Crohn's disease and the growth of para-tuberculosis bacteria. Mastitis is commonly treated with antibiotics, but the residue of antibiotics remains in the milk, increasing the likelihood of creating more antibiotic-resistant bacteria in our bodies.

rBGH in cows' blood stimulates the surplus production of another hormone called IGF-1 (Insulin-like Growth Factor-1). IGF-1 is inherently responsible for increasing milk production in both cows and humans. In addition, IGF-1 transfers to the young via the milk they drink, triggering cell growth and thus enabling the rapid growth of infants and calves. That is why IGF-1 is biologically present in mothers' milk – to help nurture their own young. However, when non-infant humans ingest cow's milk, this hormone – because it is present in the milk – still triggers rapid cell division and can thus contribute to the growth of cancer cells in the body of adults. That same concern applies, albeit to a lesser extent, even to the consumption of milk products from cows *not treated* with rBGH, including organic milk products. So it pays to be cautious about the quantities of milk products you take in. [13.6]

Note that if you read product labels carefully, you may notice a disclaimer on milk products that "no significant difference has been shown between milk derived from rBST treated and non-rBST treated cows," in apparent contradiction to the discussion here. The source of this contradiction lies in the origin of the advice – one comes from scientific studies, while the other from government-approved language on labels. As with other situations where discrepancies of advice exist, you have to decide which sources of information to honor in making your own health-related choices.

As a final point of perspective, you may buy a certain food item because of what you know about it and have tasted in it. But what else could, unexpectedly, be in that food product too? For milk produced with rBGH, specifically, it has been found that as little as 1 ml contains 1.5 million cows' white blood cells (indicating that the cow's immune system has been fighting an infection)! [13.7] Are you knowingly and willingly ingesting that?

Unnatural, poor living conditions and feed

In addition to the unnatural methods used to increase milk production for human (over)consumption, large dairy conglomerates keep cows in unnatural settings. Focused on demands for high efficiency, rapid turnaround, and bottom line profits (i.e., more cows + less space + cheap feed = more profit), dairy companies pack their cows in tiny enclosed spaces within feedlots (CAFOs), offering no opportunity to move about. This encourages animals to eat more and not expend energy, thus quickly gaining weight.

Cows are fed cheap grains (such as corn, soy, etc.), an approach that has two benefits from the standpoint of dairy companies: (a) it is more economical compared to maintaining plush green acreages for grazing or else making hay available in barns; and (b) a grain-based diet helps to rapidly fatten animals, who would be later sold for their meat. But grains (some of which are also generally engineered) are not a natural food source for cows, and this causes an inflammation of the cows' gut, requiring constant treatment with antibiotics.

Reverence for the animals has today become a thing of the past.

Conventional heavy processing of dairy

To increase shelf life, milk is processed via pasteurization or ultra-pasteurization[28], and then homogenization. Evidence suggests that milk pasteurization techniques have numerous adverse effects: denaturing delicate milk proteins; destroying enzymes; destroying vitamins C, B_{12}, and B_6; and killing beneficial bacteria, among others. In the homogenization process, in turn, pressure of up to 4000 pounds per square inch (to visualize the enormity of this, think of an elephant stepping on an ant) is applied to milk, breaking up fat molecules into multiple globules. The intent is to give milk a creamy consistency, and for the cream to not separate on the top. However, fat molecules subjected to such high pressures become oxidized and hence turn rancid. Such high temperatures and high pressures change the structure of milk, rendering it harder to break down and digest. This results in adverse health conditions, including dairy

---

[28] In the process of ultra-pasteurization, milk is heated rapidly to 280F for 2-4 seconds, then cooled instantaneously to destroy harmful microorganisms. Milk thus treated can generally stay unspoiled for months.

allergies and milk protein intolerances, which are growing rampantly in our present day society. [13.8] As you can see, the conventional milk found in most grocery stores today is nothing like what our ancestors produced and consumed.

Different practices followed by organic and smaller dairy companies

Several organic dairy companies also perform pasteurization and homogenization (as listed on product labels), but they take better care of their cows – feeding them organic (non-GMO) grains instead, and not injecting bovine growth hormones (rBGH / rBST), nor using artificial insemination techniques.

A handful of organic dairy companies and some small dairy farmers go even a step further, letting cows graze on green pastures. Some farms produce raw[29] milk from their grass-fed cows, while others vat-pasteurize[30] the milk and keep it non-homogenized, thereby preserving most of the nutrients that would have otherwise been lost under high heat and high pressure conditions.

Less processing = higher nutritive value

When cows are allowed to thrive in natural settings, the less processed their milk is, the higher its nutritive value. Milk from pasture raised or grass-fed cows is higher in nutrients, including certain anti-oxidants and heart-healthy, anti-inflammatory essential fatty acids such as ALA (alpha-linolenic acid). Grass-fed raw milk has additional benefits as it is loaded with beneficial bacteria; 60+ digestive enzymes; rich in CLA; raw fats; amino acids; vitamins A, B, C, D, E, and K; and calcium, magnesium, iron, and phosphorus. Butter from grass-fed cows' milk is rich in choline, butyric acid, vitamin K_2, and other omega-3 fatty acids that are beneficial for the heart and brain. [13.9, 13.10] Ghee (clarified butter, prepared from unsalted full fat butter) is 100% pure fat, free of milk proteins and hence ideally suited for people who need to avoid milk and its proteins. Ghee also has a high smoke point, making it suitable for

---

[29] Raw milk does not undergo any pasteurization or homogenization.
[30] In the vat-pasteurization process, milk is heated to 145F for about 30 minutes and then cooled quickly. Milk thus treated lasts for about 3 weeks under refrigeration.

cooking. Ghee prepared from grass-fed butter is rich in vitamins A, E, K_2, and also rich in CLA and butyric acid, a great immune booster. In addition to its nutritive value, ghee is also used for detoxification purposes. [13.11]

Dairy from other farming animals

Dairy is not just limited to products made from cow's milk. Goat's and sheep's milk are becoming increasingly popular, as they are more easily digested by the human body when compared to cow's milk. Both goat's and sheep's milk are lower in lactose – the main sugar contained in dairy products that some people are intolerant to. Further, the standard milk production processes associated with these animals lead to fewer concerns compared to cow's milk production.

Goat's milk is high in calcium and fatty acids. It also contains a specific type of casein, making it (as far as proteins) the closest match to human breast milk. The pH of goat's milk is similar to that of the human body, which makes it easily absorbable by our skin, keeping bacteria at bay. Goat's milk also has high levels of zinc and selenium; and nutrients like iron, calcium, phosphorus, and magnesium are more bioavailable than the ones present in cow's milk.

Sheep's milk is also higher in calcium, vitamins A, D, and E, and higher in protein. It also offers essential minerals such as zinc and magnesium. [13.12, 13.13]

Non-dairy alternatives – the good and the bad

To mitigate the problems with dairy-related allergies and intolerances, several non-dairy options have emerged. Among the more popular alternatives have been almond, rice, coconut, and soy[31] milk. Many more options of non-dairy milk have come on the market too – from quinoa, hemp, oats, cashews, hazelnuts, etc. Not only milk, but also yogurts, cheeses, butters, spreads, dressings, desserts, and other non-dairy beverages have become available. With the booming of the

---

[31] Note that soy-based products in their various forms may be problematic. If unfermented, phytoestrogens in soy mimic estrogens in the human body, hence disrupting our hormone production. Soy is also high in phytic acid, binding with useful minerals in the body, thereby preventing their absorption. Finally, non-organic soy is most likely genetically modified.

non-dairy industry lately, even here companies have been creatively offering a multitude of flavors, sweetened and unsweetened options for the growing clientele.

A few non-dairy manufacturers have been offering products with minimal processing, while the rest (even organic producers) have been using gums and thickeners, such as carrageenan, to create a milk-like, creamy consistency. Some have also been pasteurizing their non-dairy milk. All this additional processing and use of thickeners can irritate the human gut and cause digestive issues.

Feared or revered? Beneficial or not?

Milk in its purest original form is not a food to be feared, but one to be revered. It has served mankind for millennia, yielding *through alchemical processes* several different products from the one primary input – the raw milk itself. For example, cream is separated from the milk. Then the cream is churned to make butter. The butter is in turn used to make ghee (clarified butter), with its many beneficial uses. Yogurt and kefir are also derivatives of milk, naturally cultured (fermented) and unsweetened, providing our gut with a host of beneficial bacteria. Cheese, if properly cultured and aged, can also be a health food.

Remember that your *sound digestive system is fundamental* to being able to easily assimilate the benefits of pure, unprocessed (or minimally processed) organic and/or grass-fed dairy, when consumed in appropriate quantities and according to your individual constitution. Indeed, *it is possible to repair / heal your gut*, after which you can safely add back good quality dairy products, preferably unsweetened.

It is the heavy processing, the unnatural food and living conditions for the animals, the additives, and the large quantities consumed, which all combine to result in the many detrimental effects associated with dairy in our modern world.

~

One small action step you can take today: Pick a dairy product that you have not tried previously. It could be from a different dairy animal (e.g., from sheep's or goat's milk), or a minimally processed organic / grass-fed product with no added sugars. Sample a serving or two of this new dairy product for at least one day. How did you like the new dairy food when compared to your usual selections? What factors were distinctly different for you from the usual – taste, texture, smell, after-effects, and other factors? If you felt better with that new dairy product, would you be open to adding it to your regular diet or perhaps replacing one of your staples for it? Why or why not?

Need an added challenge? Eliminate all forms of dairy from your diet for three days. You may replace your usual dairy choices with minimally processed, carrageenan- and gum-free non-dairy options, or make your own non-dairy milk at home. How did your body feel upon eliminating dairy? Did you notice any changes in your digestion and elimination processes? Was there any other significant difference in how you felt without dairy? If yes, how? How did you fare with the addition of non-dairy choices to your diet? Which was your favorite, and why?

14: I was led to believe that eating fats would make me fat. But I am heavier, in spite of making a change to low-fat foods. Am I doing something wrong?

Our modern society has, over the past century, begun fragmenting and deconstructing meals into "food categories" and "nutritional elements." Instead of the simplicity and pleasant experience of plating our food and eating in joy and tranquility, many of us have been harboring doubts, fears, and confusion regarding what is on our plates. The experience of "wholeness" has gradually yielded to overwhelmingly many considerations. Our grandparents ate with the seasons and, more than likely, chose their foods intuitively, without paying as much attention to the "science" behind the foods being consumed.

Revisited: The trend toward changes in nutrition

Let us briefly revisit one of our opening questions – why has our collective outlook on food and nutrition changed so much since the days of our ancestors? A simple retort (as we have already discussed) is that both the natural and manmade ecosystems have considerably changed since the days of our ancestors. In those early days, for example, there was more biodiversity (pollinating insects, earthworms, fertile soils, and a balanced ratio of birds and animals) that supported farming practices. In contrast, in recent years the biodiversity has increasingly been under threat – mostly due to heavy industrialization, questionable farming practices, and food monopolies. This has given rise to many uncertainties and conflicting ideas that have served as an impetus for numerous scientific, governmental, and food industry bodies to research the myriad of factors related to foods, diets, and nutrients. The greater the number of inquiries and research teams, the higher the number of differing viewpoints. All these data and opinions have been driving the design and redesign of public policies around food and nutrition, thereby influencing how we relate to food (including our mealtime experiences). Meals that would have been intuitively considered well balanced are today being "sized-up," measured, and validated using external metrics. That which we once intuitively felt to be nourishing for our bodies, we have since been questioning.

The "fat" scare and its consequences

Dietary fats and, in particular, saturated fats were among the first categories of foods to be demonized by modern-day society, beginning in the 1960s. This was largely due to research by Ancel Keys, an influential physiologist, who correlated the consumption of saturated fats (e.g., butter, eggs, meats, dairy, etc.) to higher cholesterol levels and increased incidence of coronary heart disease (CHD). The low-fat advice from Keys, with blessings from policy makers, led to a notable increase in the consumption of refined carbohydrates and added sugars in place of healthy dietary fats – which in turn led to increased incidence of metabolic syndrome, characterized by a rise in triglycerides and lowering of HDL (High-Density Lipoprotein, the good cholesterol) levels. The diets of many people shifted drastically and for the worse toward a more calculated (and, more specifically, low-fat) way of eating. The processed food industry also took advantage of the low-fat fad to the detriment of its customers. Recipes were revised, replacing real butter and unrefined oils with processed margarine, vegetable shortening, and hydrogenated oils – causing a host of health issues for those who regularly consumed such foods. [14.1, 14.2]

"Fat does not make you fat" – sugar does that

By the early 1970s the English researcher John Yudkin had disproved Keys' theory, instead arguing that sugar, not saturated fats, ultimately causes CHD and high cholesterol levels. However, with much reinventing already done by the processed food industry, and a firm belief of most consumers in the validity of Ancel Keys' research findings, pointing toward sugars as the main culprit was not well received by policy makers and food manufacturers. Bringing back old-time favorite fats into the diet via traditional, wholesome foods was nearly impossible on a policy level, and the trend of consuming low-fat foods, both home-cooked and processed, continued.

In the decades since the mid-1970s (when the low-fat guidelines were issued), obesity rates have been steadily climbing worldwide. If, instead of taking to refined oils and processed foods, people had chosen to stick to eating wholesome vegetables, fruits, whole grains, and minimally processed foods (even with reduced saturated fat intake) – as their ancestors had done for generations – the rising epidemic of metabolic obesity, leading to CHD, diabetes, and other serious illnesses, may never have materialized. [14.3, 14.4]

The key takeaway is this: fat is not your "enemy," and (dietary) fat *does not* make you fat.

The "fat" dilemma

Today we have the juxtaposition where many people still religiously practice the low-fat ideology, while at the same time health advocates point in the direction of eating "real," unaltered, and wholesome fats. So we are faced with a dilemma:

1. Should we consume fats at all?
2. If yes:
   (a) How much? and
   (b) Which fats would be health promoting?

To answer these important questions, let us first understand the three types of fats.

Types of fats and their effect

- *Omega-3 fatty acids* – These have anti-inflammatory effects on the human body, and are considered most beneficial to health. Examples are fats from avocados, hemp seeds, chia seeds, organic / pastured egg yolks, raw tree nuts (e.g., pecans and macadamias), raw cocoa butter, raw dairy (or at most low-heat or vat-pasteurized), grass-fed meat, wild Alaskan salmon, sardines, and anchovies.

  These and a number of unrefined fats, such as grass-fed butter, olive oil, coconut oil, ghee, and palm fruit oil – most of which are saturated fats – are all considered *"good" fats*.

- *Omega-6 fatty acids* – These are known to have pro-inflammatory effects on the human body. They can be beneficial[32] to you if their ratio to omega-3 fatty acids in your

---

[32] If you have a cut, your immune system responds by causing temporary inflammation of the area. For this it needs the right pro-inflammatory building blocks. Once its job is done, for healing to occur, the body needs to move into an anti-inflammatory state.

diet is either 1:1 or at most 3:1. However, most people today consume these omega-6 fats in a ratio of 20:1 (and even 50:1) to omega-3's – alarmingly disproportionate! Vegetable oils (e.g., corn, canola, soybean, and sunflower), as well as some seeds and peanuts are common plant-based sources of omega-6 fatty acids. These vegetable oils are unstable under heat, converting to harmful trans-fats. (Trans-fats are also the result of a chemical change that occurs during the process of hydrogenation of vegetable oils. Products like margarine and vegetable shortening, for example, are created using the process of partial hydrogenation.) Trans-fats are the real culprits, responsible for clogging your arteries and causing heart disease, so they are among the so called *"bad" fats*. However, if you still wish to use organic vegetable oils, choose their unrefined versions and use sparingly, at low heat or raw (in salads). Since these oils are rich in omega-6 fatty acids, if you use them regularly you can create an imbalanced ratio of omega-6's to omega-3's in your body. High proportions of omega-6 fatty acids in the diet will create ripe conditions for cellular inflammation, making you susceptible to diseases such as arthritis, cardio vascular disease, diabetes, Alzheimer's, and cancer, among others. Due to unregulated amounts of processed foods and cheap fast (junk) foods proliferating in modern societies, it is rather easy to "overdose" on omega 6's, so beware!

Note that both omega-3 and omega-6 are considered *essential fatty acids* (EFAs) – they are not produced by the body, and hence must be acquired through food sources.

- *Omega-9 fatty acids* – These are naturally produced in the human body (hence considered "non-essential"), if there is a sufficient amount of omega-3's and omega-6's.

For normal growth and development of your body, a balance of all three types of fatty acids is needed. [14.5]

Why "good" fats are so crucial?
Consuming "good" fats brings many benefits. Most notable among them are:

- providing optimal fuel for your brain and heart – both systems crucially depend on it;

- increasing satiety;

- providing proper building blocks for your cell membranes and hormones;

- helping lower your body's cholesterol levels – contrary to popular myths and misconceptions;

- aiding mineral absorption (e.g., calcium);

- catalyzing the conversion of carotene to vitamin A;

- being a proper carrier for important fat soluble vitamins: A, D, E, and K;

- preventing cancers;

- acting as antiviral agents.

Conversely, not receiving enough healthy omega-3 fats via your diet can result in conditions such as: weight gain, allergies, arthritis, dry hair, dry skin, brittle nails, poor concentration, poor sleep, depression, brain fog, memory problems, and fatigue. [14.6]

The saturated fat and cholesterol myth
For decades, saturated fat and cholesterol have been wrongly vilified as primary triggers for heart disease. As you have seen from the above discussion, unrefined saturated fats (along with other good fats) are *essential* for your body's optimum functioning. Cholesterol, too, is not only beneficial but also required in your body. It helps in the production of hormones, vitamin D, cell membranes, and bile acids, among many other crucial functions. [14.7]

There are two types of cholesterol: LDL (Low-Density Lipoprotein) and HDL (High-Density Lipoprotein). LDL is considered "bad" cholesterol, responsible for clogging up the arteries. HDL, on the other hand, is considered "good" cholesterol that is supportive of heart health, removing excess arterial plaque. Consuming "good" fats increases the level of HDL; "bad" fats contribute to a rise of LDL levels. [14.8]

Blood cholesterol levels are measured via a "Lipid Profile" blood test. The components typically measured are: LDL, HDL, triglycerides (TGL), and total cholesterol. Most cholesterol tests, as done in hospital labs today, take only these four individual markers into account when calculating the risk of heart disease. There are other, often better, indicators of heart disease risk, which are not considered in the standard lab tests: markers such as VLDL (Very Low-Density Lipoprotein), Lipoprotein A, the ratios of some of these markers, etc. Two important ratios to consider from your own "Lipid profile" test are: (a) HDL/total cholesterol (24% and above is ideal, while less than 10% is indicative of significant heart disease risk), and (b) TGL/HDL (below 2 is ideal). [14.9]

How much "good" dietary fat do you need?
There are many conflicting schools of thought, each suggesting certain "ideal" amounts for maintaining good health. To give you some perspective, the National Institutes of Health (NIH) recommends that adults consume 20%-35% of all daily calories from fats, and respectively 25%-35% for children above age 4. The recommendation by USDA for saturated fats, in particular, is to keep those at less than 10% of daily calories. Most alternative and holistic health practitioners, in contrast, suggest that 50%-70% of your daily calories come from good fats. [14.10]

Once again, consider your individual constitution when choosing the appropriate amount *for you*. If you are unsure, consult a health care professional whom you trust.

Note that in a few specific instances consuming a regular amount of "good" fats may be detrimental. One such (temporary or long-term) condition is when the body has difficulty metabolizing fats. When its primary energy source, glucose, has been expended, a healthy functioning body will digest fats to get energy. Inability to do so would halt bodily processes, so for people with fatty acid metabolism disorder or liver disorders must maintain healthy blood glucose levels and eat a low-fat diet. [14.11]

~

One small action step you can take today: For one day, commit to eating all your meals without "considerations" or harboring any doubts about what is on your plate. Give yourself permission to eat your traditional cultural favorites, made lovingly with wholesome ingredients, including "good" fats – ones that your great grandmother would recognize! Strive to use methods of preparation that your ancestors also used. You may invite others of like mind to join you for one or all meals. How did it feel bringing old traditions back into your life? How different was this mealtime experience, stepping out of your comfort zone and not having to use external metrics to "size-up" your plate?

Need an added challenge? Take an inventory of your pantry and set aside those pre-packaged foods that contain omega-6 fatty acids and trans-fats (e.g., if the nutrition label says, partially hydrogenated / margarine / shortening). What percentage of foods in your household is laden with omega-6's and trans-fats? Did the results surprise you, and if so, how? Check to see if one or more of the symptoms (listed above), corresponding to not getting enough beneficial omega-3's, applies to you? Could these symptoms (or lack thereof) be somehow connected with your regular diet? What foods are you willing to add to your diet to help provide additional beneficial omega-3's? How do you believe your symptoms, if any, might change with more beneficial fats in your diet?

15: How do I find good quality foods in a store?

To properly answer this question, one has to start with *awareness* of what is beneficial (good quality) versus what can be harmful (poor quality) — a topic that some previous questions have touched on.

The next step is to find out what is inside a food item that you think of buying. This is made easier by the attached *nutritional label* to most food products, except fresh produce. [15.1] Note that this type of nutritional information from a label is not available at many restaurants yet, so ensuring good quality there is generally harder. For example, restaurant menus in the United States are not required to disclose ingredients such as salt and sugar content, the presence of artificial colors or flavors, the sources of the ingredients of a given dish, etc.

What to pay attention to

For *fresh produce*, look for:
    (1) whether it has been organically or conventionally grown; and
    (2) the location where it has been grown.
This much is often being disclosed in grocery stores.

For all *packaged (non-fresh) food products*, look at the following on the product packaging label:
    (1) the list of ingredients, and for each ingredient identify:
        (a) if it is listed as being organically grown (if not, it likely has been conventionally grown);
        (b) if you generally recognize and would expect to see this ingredient (e.g., added sugars in non-dessert foods can be suspicious);
        (c) if it is among a few allergenic ingredients you might be sensitive to;
        (d) if it is from a list of commonly known food-like "offenders."
    (2) the expiration date for the product;
    (3) the geographical location where the food was produced. (This information is sometimes, but not always, available on packages.)

(4) the company-producer – it may give you clues based on any prior history you are aware of;

(5) the type of packaging – certain types may be harmful (see below).

Doing such scanning and screening of ingredients becomes more effective as you gain experience, and technological applications (apps on mobile phones) may simplify the task. [15.2]

Now for a brief explanation about how some of the above factors matter:

Organic vs. conventional
The difference between organically and conventionally grown items, generally, comes down to:

- whether pesticides and herbicides (i.e., harmful chemicals) have been used to control weeds and pests. The organic food standard prohibits the use of synthetic pesticides and herbicides, whereas conventionally-grown foods almost certainly imply the heavy use of such harmful chemicals. "The dirty dozen" [15.3] is a notorious list of conventionally grown fruits and vegetables that have very high levels of pesticide residue – something to be avoided whenever possible. In contrast, "the clean fifteen" is a similar list of produce with low levels of pesticide residue [15.4] – signifying a potentially good choice (except for papaya and corn, which may be genetically modified – see below) if your budget does not allow purchasing the organic counterpart item or if the organic option is not available.

- whether other artificial chemicals have been incorporated to stimulate growth (e.g., hormones and antibiotics injected to milk-producing cows) or to preserve freshness (e.g., petroleum-based wax put on apples). Again, the organic food standard prohibits such chemicals from the food supply.

- whether the product has been genetically modified – a controversial technological process whereby different species are being combined at the gene level to create something new that does not exist in Nature, with unknown and potentially hazardous health consequences to the consumer. Certain food items are virtually guaranteed to have been genetically modified, if they are not listed as either "organic" or "non-GMO" on the product label, and especially if grown in the US. Watch out for soy-based and corn-based products, as well as strawberries, canola, Hawaiian papaya, cottonseed, alfalfa, and others.

Allergenic ingredients
The list of allergenic ingredients is short and typically well known to people who are aware of having allergies toward certain foods. Note that some of the items on this list are generally considered harmless, and may be quite safe to consume for people without existing allergies toward them. At the same time, it is quite safe to omit such items from your menu, if you are unsure.

The list of known common allergens includes: gluten (present in many popular grains and flours), dairy, eggs, soy, corn, peanuts, tree nuts, and shellfish. There may be other allergens too, specific to an individual's digestive system – hence the importance of knowing yourself and choosing appropriately.

Food-like "offenders"
All items in this category are unnaturally processed (chemically or genetically) and harmful to humans. Some are known carcinogens, and all have poor consequences to our health and wellness. The list includes:

Types of food "offenders"	Examples
artificial flavors, natural[33] flavors	MSG (monosodium glutamate – a chemical), table salt (purely sodium chloride, NaCl, devoid of other minerals), etc.
artificial colors	red 40, blue 1, yellow 5, etc.

---

[33] Note that the use of the term "natural" is not regulated in the US when it comes to foods, so the presence of this word on a product label does not necessarily imply what the word usually means. It is commonly used for marketing reasons.

Types of food "offenders"	Examples
preservatives	potassium sorbate, sodium benzoate, or even added sodium
artificial sweeteners	high-fructose corn syrup, aspartame (a.k.a. E981), maltose, dextrose, maltodextrin, saccharin, beet sugar, etc.
food "enhancers"	generally listed with "E" followed by a 3-digit number, e.g., E321, E981
trans-fats[34]	margarine, (partially) hydrogenated oils, vegetable shortening

By staying up-to-date on health and nutrition-related news, over time you will start recognizing more offending items and thus be equipped to avoid them. Such updating and upgrading of your knowledge is important since a number of these offenders have been identified as likely carcinogens, but have not yet been banned (in most countries) from entering the food system. [15.5, 15.6, 15.7, 15.8] See §26 for some reliable sources of information.

Location of production

The reason why a product's location may matter is related to the respective environment and process of production. For example, rice grown in India, Pakistan, or California is known to contain much less arsenic (a harmful chemical present in irrigation waters used in the production process for rice) compared to rice grown elsewhere, and therefore the former kind is preferable health-wise.

With experience, this label scanning process will become easier, faster, and a natural thing you do whenever you pick up an item at the store and consider whether to buy it. While this process was unnecessary prior to the advent of the modern industrialized agriculture, today it is increasingly important as a preemptive measure of protection for maintaining good health.

---

[34] Trans-fats are the product of refining/hydrogenating oils. Be sure they are listed as 0g on the nutritional label. They are also prohibited from the food supply in certain locations.

Type of packaging

Certain types of packaging may transfer harmful molecules into the food on contact. Examples include: BPA[35]/BPS-lined containers (many cans, polycarbonate bottles #7), soft plastics (especially #1, #3, and #6), lead[36]-based crystal (commonly used for glassware), aluminum foil (especially under high temperature), etc. [15.9]

~

One small action step you can take today: Get curious about product labels. Next time you go grocery shopping, take some time to read the ingredients list and nutrition label of the items you normally buy, as well as of some items you do not usually purchase. Are there ingredients you do not recognize? Later read up more on those strange sounding names (you may choose to navigate some website links we have listed under §26). Would your grandmother or great grandmother recognize those ingredients? Are you open and willing to replace questionable items, after your research, with "cleaner" ones? Why or why not?

Need an added challenge? For one week, commit to buying and ingesting only foods that are made with 5 ingredients or fewer. Also ensure that the ingredients listed are those that your predecessors might easily recognize. When unsure, such as when dining at a restaurant, ask (e.g., the waiter or chef) for details on ingredients that are present in the dish you wish to order. Reflect upon your experience of becoming a "food detective" for a week. Do you feel empowered in advocating for your own needs or constrained? If yes, how? How do you think your body will respond in the long run to the kind of foods you consumed for that week, compared to your usual diet?

---

[35] Bisphenol-A (a.k.a., BPA) is also found in the paper used for printing receipts in most stores. Be sure to wash hands well after handling.
[36] Lead and other harmful heavy metals (featured in the so called "California 65 proposition" warnings on products) are commonly found in electronics equipment, including cables, cell phone and computer screens, chargers, etc. Thoroughly and promptly wash hands after handling, and definitely do not eat while handling (a frequent habit of cell phone users).

16: What if I do not, or cannot, eat a healthy diet?

"Life happens," as the saying goes. On occasion you may not have access to healthful foods – such as at a social gathering or while on the road. Minor digressions and "offenses" are not as problematic, because the human body is equipped to recharge and rebuild itself. Instead, it is the chronic, regular lack of care and the exposure to unhealthy substances that hurts the most.

Cultivating sound habits

If you wish to change a poor habit (e.g., one that hurts your health) or to create a new positive habit, it all starts with *awareness* (of where you are currently and where you wish to direct your energies); a firm intent; and practical knowledge of what and how to do; and then actually doing it. This handbook can be helpful in all dimensions.

When it comes to eating habits, it is important to cultivate knowledge about why some foods may be more beneficial (respectively, more damaging) than others. You will be empowered to make better food choices if:

- you understand how food is often processed these days – using industrial oils and other chemical additives and preservatives; and

- you are aware of available healthy alternatives for snacks and meals.

Practical healthy alternatives at home and away

At home:

- For a crunchy texture, instead of potato chips (often fried or baked with trans-fats or poor-quality oils[37], and depleted of nutrients), consider kale chips (usually baked or dehydrated),

---

[37] Poor-quality oils include those that are unstable at higher temperatures and become easily oxidized and rancid, contributing to heart disease. Also, canola oil, corn oil, soybean oil, and cottonseed oil are commonly derived from genetically engineered ingredients. Preferable are avocado oil and coconut oil.

carrots, celery (organic only, to avoid the "dirty dozen" list; and cooked, to remove compounds that over-sensitize the skin to ultraviolet radiation), or seaweed (organic and sourced from waters outside of the Pacific Ocean, due to concerns about radiation exposure from Fukushima).

- For protein, instead of hamburgers and pizzas, opt for nuts, nut butters, hummus (i.e., mainly mashed garbanzo beans), or boiled eggs.

- For additional ideas, see the resources in [16.1].

At restaurants:

- Choose among the menu options that best represent a healthy meal, based on your knowledge.

- If you are able, patronize restaurants serving organic food, or at least ones that have options for local and sustainable items.

- You may always ask a restaurant to prepare your meal *customized* to your preferences (e.g., using olive oil instead of vegetable oil; pan-seared fish instead of fried fish; etc.).

- Choose dishes with fewer ingredients, such as salads, rice and beans, and steamed or grilled vegetables.

The true cost of food
On a personal level, some people cite higher costs as a deterrent to enjoying nutritious foods on a daily basis. But their intended "savings" from consuming cheap food are often both unreal and unwise. The poor quality of foods they choose hurts their bodies – leading to inferior quality of life, frequent doctor visits, and increased use of prescription medicines. To cater to unnatural cravings they also likely seek more fast foods. In the end, the person spends manifold the amount they had "saved."

On a larger scale, the industry that pushes cheap food has standard practices that result in: increased pollution and environmental degradation; poor workers' conditions at factories and in fast food chains; low attention to food quality; disregard for fair trade practices; and employment of child labor in developing countries.

These examples illustrate the classic case of overemphasis on short-term savings that leads to extensive long-term damage: both personal to the consumer, and societal to all of us.

If your budget or habits truly do not allow you to switch over (to more nutritious foods) fully, you can always instead take small but regular steps – one little change at a time. Pay attention to the newly found results you get along the way, and make incremental progress as you feel guided to.

A path toward steady improvement

Once you start eating healthful foods more often, your body will more readily receive the necessary nutrients and will feel "balanced" much of the time. In turn, your desire for less healthy and less natural foods will diminish.

You are *the master of your body, and the master of yourself!* You do not have to be a slave to anyone or anything:

- Not to your taste buds. After all, who is boss – you or your taste buds?

- Not to food marketers and the dictates of the processed food industry. Their interests for short-term quick profitability often do not align with your interests for long-term good health.

- Not to doctors and health insurance companies. Do you remember what glowing health feels like? Did they ever sell you on the (wrong) idea that your health is supposed to steadily deteriorate as you age, and that prescription medicines and invasive treatments are required to stay afloat?

- Not to rationally-sounding skeptics among family and friends. Expect them to disagree with any changes you undertake, so just do what you need to do without much fanfare. When they see your results, they may reconsider their initial positions or even ask you quietly for advice.

Self-discipline becomes effortless, rather than grim, once you put the "right fuel" inside your body. Your thinking becomes clearer, your body feels more vitality, and you cannot help but treat yourself with utmost care. Just as a car runs more efficiently when you give it the right kind of fuel, so will your body.

When you eat right by honoring your individual constitution, you will feel far better overall – perhaps better than you even imagine it possible (especially if you have been on the ill-health treadmill for long). You will also not need to visit a doctor as often. You will not eat junk foods to curb cravings, and your body will need *less* food overall to get the proper nutrition it needs. As a result, you would also save money in the long run. Health is indeed wealth, quite literally! May your path be blessed and successful!

~

One small action step you can take today: For one week, replace your regular crunchy snacks (if they include deep fried items and/or ones made with trans-fats / hydrogenated oils or other fake fats) with healthier crunchy snacks, such as those listed above or in the references. How did you feel, replacing your regular "go to" snacks with new healthier ones? Did you observe any changes in your cravings and/or energy levels and moods?

Need an added challenge? For three weeks, whenever you go to eat at a restaurant or pick up food from a deli, make sure that your food is "clean" and made to the specifications described above. Speak to your waiter or chef, as needed, to ensure that your personal dietary needs are fully met. How did you like the experience of advocating for yourself? How did you feel about the restaurant's / deli's willingness to offer you a personalized meal? Reflect upon your experiences.

17: How much and how often does it serve me well to eat? I find myself hungry often...

Key influencing factors

It is commonly believed that how much you eat at a time depends on:

- your appetite (which is the expressed need for fresh biochemical energy to enter your system);

- the amount of food your stomach can comfortably hold (typically, the size of your clenched fist).

Other, less well acknowledged factors that influence how much you eat are:

- the nutrient density of the food;

- the time of day (or night);

- your emotional state;

- your mental state;

- stress level (including physical stress);

- cravings;

- any eating disorders;

- cultural upbringing;

- existing habits;

- your own conscious choice; and

- the level of mindfulness (versus compulsiveness) in attending to your needs.

Appetite

Momentary stress levels can inflate or deflate your appetite. Chronic stress, on the other hand, can create a "blind spot": you become so entrenched in that state of stress that it becomes a part of you that you are no longer able to see as separate. Then you are no longer experiencing stress as an external stimulus; rather, you have become one with it. Stressors often lead to chemical and hormonal imbalances in the body and its endocrine system, in turn impacting your emotions, mind state, and from there your appetite also. They can affect how much you eat, when you eat, and also what you eat.

Cravings

Food cravings, similarly, influence what and when you eat, besides how much you eat. Several factors induce cravings, including dehydration, mineral imbalances, and even cultural background. Cravings are a messenger for what your body needs in that moment. So instead of feeling guilty about a craving, tune in and ask your body what it needs. (See the action step below.)

Very often, cravings for something sweet may be a sign of thirst; so a glass of water may be your best "prescription" in that moment. Likewise, craving salty foods may indicate experiencing a mineral imbalance. If you suddenly start craving foods from your childhood (that you now normally do not eat), then you are likely either feeing homesick or desiring a (re)connection with a loved one, the memory of whom is rekindled as you think about that particular food.

Who is boss?

Whether it be due to stress, cravings, or any other influence, it is important to also understand that eating per se is a personal choice. The question then to ask is, "Who is the boss?" Are you (as the boss) empowered to make conscious choices for yourself, or are you "playing victim" to your circumstances? What to eat, how much to eat, and when to eat are mostly under *your control*, except if there is a diagnosed eating disorder (e.g., anorexia, bulimia, etc.) or any trauma adversely impacting your ability to make sound choices. For example, at mealtime if you stop eating *before* you are completely full – just at the point when it feels most tempting to continue – the food you have eaten will be processed by your body quite efficiently. More often than not, people take in several bites even after they are 100% full, as the stomach has received a skewed perception of the brain's satiation signal. There can be several reasons for this: eating too quickly[38] (which also implies not chewing the food well[39]), or not

---

[38] As a practical tip, imagine sitting for an hour-long formal meal (though you do not have to take 1 hour in reality). Since you will have to be present for the full hour, it is best to pace yourself and not gulp down the food in

recognizing the point at which to stop (for this, training with conscious awareness can help, over time), or having a weak will.

How important are calories, really?
Calories are a very popular and often misunderstood term. They represent the amount of biochemical energy packed in a given food product. While that caloric number matters (e.g., too many or too few calories in the food will lead to imbalances in the human organism), other factors are just as important in the choice of what to eat for your energy needs.

Among these qualitative factors are:

- *The actual source of the food* – A bag of pretzel chips contains approximately the same number of calories as an apple, but the nutritive value of these two foods differs significantly.

- *The nutrient density of the food* – Which meal would you rather eat: two tablespoons of spirulina and hemp seeds, or a plateful of various greens, vegetables, and some protein with an olive oil dressing? One is not always better than the other. Most people are conditioned to experience better satiety with the "volume" of food containing balanced nutrition, as opposed to a super-food charged with balanced multi-nutrients but hardly any volume. Even if the number of calories is the same, the food that has more volume tends to appeal more. This is in part due to the inherent desire for mastication (chewing) that humans have. Therefore, you can sprinkle "super-nutrients" into your regular healthy meal to boost its nutritive value, while your body gets satiated as you spend time chewing food. Some nutrient-dense foods that also pack sufficient volume and are easily satiating are: walnuts, eggs, kale, and beans, among others.

- *The mechanism of deriving calories from food* – There are two

---

the first few minutes, only to sit in front of empty plates while others around you savor their meals for the rest of the hour.
[39] It is recommended to chew each bite you take in at least 20 times before you swallow it. This allows the enzymes in your saliva – they are there for this reason – to pre-digest the food, making it easier on your stomach.

complementary mechanisms the body uses to get energy. One mechanism converts food into glucose, storing any leftovers as fat in our cells. This fat is the reserve source of fuel that drives the other mechanism, in which the stored fat is burned for energy. For long-term wellbeing you must derive your calories via both mechanisms.

Our hunter-gatherer ancestors did not have a constant daily supply of breakfast, lunch, dinner, and a few snacks in between. It was often a feast or a famine for them. So humans evolved with a genetic predisposition to be able to live even without eating regularly. It was due to the steady energy derived from burning fat (stored in fat cells). Our bodies were literally designed to make energy last through less (and less frequent) food intake.

The modern way of life (and nutrition) is often quite different, driven primarily by frequently taking in new food, which the body metabolizes as glucose and uses for its energy needs. This calorie-deriving mechanism uses glucose, which has a "roller coaster" quality – peaking quickly then crashing down. That is not sustainable for good health in the long term.

If you over-utilize this glucose-based mechanism, you would not give your body the rest needed to trigger the fat-burning mechanism. Thus, the fat stored in your cells will not be used up, resulting in weight gain and "stubborn weight." Also, over time your body will become glucose-dependent for its energy, making it seem to you as if there is no other possible energy source to reach for. But you can always train your body to revert back to its natural inclination of utilizing both mechanisms in a balanced way.

To use an analogy, when you give a system (even a machine) rest time, its longevity improves[40]. Similarly, when you give your digestive system some rest – including by spacing out meals and by offering it nutrient-dense foods – your body will not need to work as hard or as often to break down a larger quantity of food, and hence your health outcome would likely be improved too. [17.1]

---

[40] In lab tests on animals, it was established that a lower-calorie diet was associated with improved longevity.

Without nutrient-dense foods, your body will give you signals of imbalance. If you attempt to satiate it by eating foods that have "empty" calories (e.g., junk foods), you will likely not receive the needed nutrients, and you may consume a larger quantity to compensate for the lack. In the end, the popular adage "a calorie is a calorie" does not prove to be correct.

Beware of serving sizes – how much?
Generally speaking, a standard serving size visually corresponds to food that comfortably fits (i.e., is not piled up) on a standard plate (approx. 9-10 inches in diameter) and consists of nutritious items from all major food groups (i.e., complex carbohydrates, proteins, fibers, vitamins and minerals, and fats). It often includes some grain, vegetables, animal or plant proteins, and some oil / fat (e.g., olive oil, ghee, or butter). Your individual serving size can vary depending on: how nutrient-dense your food is; the volume it packs; how you combine foods; your hunger level; as well as your age, gender, current activity level, etc.

That said, serving sizes are not standardized, so food manufacturers sometimes manipulate them in order to make their products appear better on the nutritional labels than they actually are. (For example, a cup of a certain drink may contain 20 grams of added sugars, so to claim a "low-sugar" quality on the package, the product manufacturer may list the serving size as ¼ cup, thus having only 5 grams of sugar per serving, seemingly low-sugar. But are you normally drinking ¼ cup or more?) So be sure to pay attention to the serving size as well on the label, particularly how realistic that amount may be for your typical meal.

Number of meals
To determine how many meals per day are appropriate for you, honor your individual constitution and lifestyle. Do not blindly follow rules or other people's habits, including the time honored, "3 square meals a day" or "6 small meals a day" concepts. Take into consideration your unique needs. Over time, as you continue to make conscious food choices, eating nutrient-dense foods and following the cues that your body is giving you, you may find that you require fewer meals a day and/or a smaller quantity in order to

feel satisfied and energized. Here again, there is *no "magic number"* for how many meals to eat. Let your conscious awareness help you get trained in eating mindfully and in a relaxed state, consuming nutritious foods, hence allowing your body, mind, and spirit to continue to guide you.

The importance of timing

Not all times of the day are created equal. Digestion and assimilation are most effective during certain time windows. Hence it is commonly recommended to eat your main meals during those periods – often mornings and afternoons or early evenings. [17.2] Chronic late-night eating may adversely impact your metabolism, hence your sleep cycles, as well as other biomarkers (e.g., blood pressure, blood sugar, lipid profile, etc.).

The type of food and the time of its consumption also impact your blood sugar level. Regularly driving that level high is known to be detrimental to optimal health: such spikes in blood sugar may lead to chronic diseases such as diabetes. You can counteract or avoid such spikes by:

- *pairing high-glycemic foods with low-glycemic* [17.3], e.g., sprinkling lemon or vinegar on baked potatoes (which otherwise would be prone to drive the blood sugar levels high);

- *taking in foods that are not exclusively sweet*, or at least not eating them in large quantities at a time (e.g., being careful with ice cream).

∼

One small action step you can take today: For the next three days, while eating a meal, check in with yourself frequently to see if you are feeling satiated yet. When you find yourself feeling compelled to take in one more serving (or even one more bite), not so much because you are still hungry, but because of past conditioning, then please put your fork down and exercise your will to stop eating. Notice how you feel in about 20 minutes, when your body's satiation signals will have caught up. Are you still hungry? What else is your body trying to tell you? Do you have more (or less) energy through the rest of the day leading up to your next meal? Why do you believe this is so?

Need an added challenge? Become the "Boss" for a week! Closely monitor your hunger cues, cravings, default eating habits, thirst, and other factors associated with your daily nourishment through food. Ask yourself this question (when observing these factors), "Dear body of mine, do you have a genuine need for [state what it is] in order to feel nurtured in this moment?" If you "hear" (intuitively, as a subtle bodily response) a 'yes', then go ahead and take in what it is that your body asks for. If the answer feels more like a 'no', then inquire further, "What do you truly require in this moment to feel nurtured?" Offer yourself that "gift" in this moment. How did you feel engaging in a dialog with your body? What did you learn from this experience?

18: Do I really need to drink water besides what is in food and other beverages? I do not feel thirsty as often...

Just over 70% of the Earth's surface is covered by water. Approximately 70% of your body by weight is water content. This is not a random coincidence of numbers; there is a deep interrelationship of harmony between the human body and its habitat, and between the functioning of the planetary system and of the human body system. Just as the Earth has a crucial water cycle of evaporation and re-hydration, so has your body. Altering the water balance of either will alter its nature and workings. You need to *maintain that balance* in order to properly function internally.

Hydration factors

The term *hydration* refers to the method for restoring water balance in the body, dissolving toxins, and flushing out by-products of digestion. Proper hydration depends on several factors:

- *Quantity* – how much you drink. This is what most of the popular recommendations focus on, but it is only one of several crucial factors.

- *Quality* – what specifically you drink. Water can come from different sources, with different concentrations of minerals, potential presence of pollutants, etc.

- *Timing* – when you drink. The result is not the same if you drink before versus after a meal, before going to sleep versus after awakening, etc.

- *Channel* – how you take in hydration: directly through the mouth, or absorbed through the skin (e.g., when soaked, while showering), etc.

Quantity – How much to drink

There are many schools of thought regarding how much water one ought to drink for optimal functioning of the body. Some proclaim that drinking 8 glasses of water per day is vital for you (that sounds quite simple), while others recommend that you drink more (and still others – less) in order to help "flush" your system daily. It is important, however, to reckon that *what works well for one person may not be suitable for another.* It is a good idea to take into consideration your own unique body constitution, activity level, age, weight, local weather, and so on, before determining your own "magic" number for the ideal quantity of water to take in.

Here are some alternative ideas to consider, with our brief practical comments on each. Note that some of these popular recommendations do not fit well with others. See which one(s) *resonate best with you* and your individual needs:

- "Drink only to thirst, and a little bit more." Since your body sends you signals of all kinds constantly, paying attention to and following such hints will help you over time to become more and more in tune with your internal workings – an additional priceless benefit of that strategy. Furthermore, your body is equipped, through evolution, to deal with a temporary water shortage internally – but it is not similarly equipped to deal with water overprovision, so avoid sipping water constantly if you are not thirsty. [18.1] The caveat here is if you are undergoing a cleanse / detox, a fast, or any energy healing, then for the duration of these processes it is recommended to drink more water than your usual.

- Drink less water (and less frequently) if you are consuming many foods that are rich in water, such as watermelon, lettuce, and soups. The value here is that this strategy takes into account also the specificity of your food intake.

- Drink half of your ideal body weight in ounces per day (e.g., if your ideal weight is 120 lbs., drink 60 oz.). This may be excessive, since it does not take into account your food intake, nor any other parameter of your unique body constitution – all in favor of simplicity of calculation.

- Look at the typical color of your urine. If it is very dark yellow, then you need to drink more water to help your body flush out. If it is colorless, then you likely have over-consumed water. And if the color is pale yellow then your water intake is likely on track. Drinking too little water may over time lead to dehydration and toxins building up inside of you, as salts cannot be properly dissolved. Drinking too much may instead lead to mineral deficiencies over time, as vital minerals get flushed out of your system along with excess water. So experiment, observe, and optimize your intake based on the personalized feedback that your urine color gives you. And, of course, pee when your body sends you that signal, to help release unnecessary material quickly, and to deepen your attunement to your inner signals.

In our present day, with technology allowing you to alter the weather in your living spaces with devices for climate control such as furnaces and air conditioners, your innate senses are bound to get confused between what the weather feels like outdoors versus what the body experiences in the artificially created indoor environment (which dominates many people's daily lives). This discrepancy also impacts your thirst cues. For example, in hot summer months when you would otherwise naturally feel more thirsty (perhaps due to increased perspiration) and hence be inclined to drink more water, you may in actuality drink much less if you stayed indoors with the air conditioner turned on, as you may not feel as thirsty (perhaps due to less perspiration). If, however, you choose to spend more time in places where your body is naturally in harmony with the external environment as is, without manmade "alterations," you will be better off following your natural thirst cues as they would be a good guide to what your system truly needs in that moment. This discussion merits reiterating that when you attune your inner nature to Mother Nature, you open up to experiencing greater harmony and balance in your body, mind, and spirit.

Quality – What to drink
Fresh water is by far the best-known *hydrating* drink. In modern times, however, many people consume various other fluids and beverages in substantial quantities: sodas, pasteurized juices, teas, coffees, energy drinks, milk, alcohol, etc. Several of these are known to *actually dehydrate* – rather than hydrate – the body, and many beverages are laden with caffeine and/or sugar. So it is important to include only those fluids (besides water) that are hydrating, nourishing, and free of chemical additives (including artificial sweeteners and colors) and much sugar. Some choices for such healthier hydrating alternatives are: coconut water, Kombucha[41],

freshly squeezed vegetable and fruit juices, some herbal teas, and unsweetened milk (dairy or non-dairy), among others.

Fresh water quality

"Water, water everywhere, but not a drop to drink" is a well-known quote. It is a fact (at the time of this writing) that ~71% of the Earth's surface is water. Of the known available water resources on our planet 96.5% is saltwater and the remaining 3.5% is fresh water. [18.2] Most land creatures, including humans, depend on sharing these 3.5% fresh water sources for survival.

Yet the integrity of most (if not all) water sources on Earth has been compromised to some degree. Our waters (and air) are being polluted daily as a result of by-products and run-offs from various industries; toxic gas emissions; pesticides and fertilizers from agriculture; toxic sludge draining into rivers and oceans; etc. The fresh water intended for human consumption is often heavily treated with chemicals such as chlorine to help kill off germs and other pathogens before reaching us through faucets. This treatment process removes most of the heavier particles of industrial toxicity and sludge along with pathogenic bacteria. However, through this process, chemicals such as chlorine and fluoride make their way into the "treated" water, in addition to chemical residues such as arsenic, antibiotics, etc., that do not get removed during treatment, thereby entering our bodies and causing harm in higher concentrations. [18.3] Therefore, it is vitally important to have the awareness of how you can obtain clean water for consumption. It would serve you well to request a water quality assessment for your locale / neighborhood.

Your body is ~70% water, your brain has even higher (85%) water content, and the rest is in the muscle tissues of the body. So be mindful of how you replenish and manage the quality of this vitally important resource inside of you by choosing wisely. [18.4] Below we list some ideas that may help you to make informed and wise practical choices for obtaining clean water to meet your needs. It is important to note that the field has a lot more to offer than most

---

[41] A naturally fermented fizzy drink, with a tiny amount of alcohol. Kombucha, like other fermented foods and drinks, promotes good digestion.

people are even aware of. The topic of drinking water quality and access to water resources is often ill-addressed at the public health level, and some of the promising approaches have not been studied for comparison of their effectiveness:

- *using collected rainwater* (in areas without much air pollution) – avoids the harm from chemical treatment in the first place, though bacteria and remnants from industrial pollution may be present to some degree;

- *using water from nearby natural springs and wells* – can be inexpensive, but the water source needs to be tested (e.g., public health departments can run water quality tests), since even natural springs may be polluted due to industrial activity that affects underground aquifers (e.g., oil fracking and pushing wastewater back into the ground);

- *boiling water and keeping it in a clean container* – removes pathogens and is one of the cheapest options to improve on the quality of tap water;

- *procuring a carbon filter with a dispenser* – helps in removing some harmful substances such as asbestos, Giardia cyst (a parasite), lead, certain pesticides, trihalomethanes, copper, mercury, cadmium, volatile organic compounds (VOCs), and reducing chlorine (odor and taste) and zinc;

- *installing* advanced *water filters* – removes most of the chemical additives and impurities in tap water [18.5, 18.6], and can be installed per faucet / shower head or for the entire home at the source;

- *using a reverse osmosis or a steam distillation water purification system* (at home or at a nearby health store) – offers one of the best purification qualities attainable on a mass scale by removing even the toughest chemical additives;

- *keeping water in copper containers* – helps to rapidly purify and energize water;

- *making alkalized / ionized water* – helps in maintaining the pH balance of your body, and contains high levels of anti-oxidants [18.7, 18.8];

- *making structured water* – helps to purify and energize water at the level of its physical structure, beyond what chemical filters can achieve [18.9];

- *blessing and shaking water* – alters the physical / structural properties of water, and purifies it by clearing its "memory" [18.1, 18.10, 18.11];

- *purchasing purified / distilled bottled water* – obtains purified water without a large upfront investment in a purification system, but still comes at a price (~$1/gallon, though much less than coffee!). If water is kept in plastic bottles for a long time, harmful chemicals (BPA, BPS, etc.) may leach and negatively impact the human endocrine system (e.g., pituitary gland, thyroid gland, adrenal gland, etc.); plus, plastic bottles require recycling facilities which are not universally present.

What explains the "magic" of water?
Conventional science, dominated by outdated notions in chemistry, sees water as a molecule with very simple properties. The mainstream still does not recognize water's ability to hold memory (of what it has been through) via different spatial orientations of the molecule's atoms, as well as between multiple water molecules. Recent scientific discoveries give evidence that water can indeed have much more complex behaviors. [18.10, 18.11, 18.12, 18.13]

The human body in its pristine state can be viewed as a repository of negatively charged water. In an environment of positive charges (acidic, low pH) a person grows tired quickly. So the body's innate intelligence aims to restore and rejuvenate the body by maximizing its negative charges and getting rid of positive charges through exhalation, sweat, and urination (all of which are acidic, low pH).

Drinking alkalized water, breathing deeply near a waterfall or at the seaside, and walking barefoot all help to accomplish this – they aid our health and also feel good. Walking barefoot, in particular, is healthful partly due to the powerful electric field of the negatively charged Earth (~100 V/m near the Earth's surface), inducing "fourth-phase water" – an intermediate phase between liquid water and solid ice [18.12, 18.13] – inside the human body. The same is the effect of drinking water from just-melted ice (as advised by some ancient cultures): it is fourth-phase water, rich in charged molecules and thus often referred to as "living water." Turbulence (e.g., by shaking the water or via the effect of ocean waves) builds fourth-phase water too.

As human organisms, we get our energy partly from light (especially infrared light, which is ubiquitous and readily absorbed by the body) interacting with the water inside. The light splits water molecules and thus creates a battery effect inside our bodies. This explains the energizing feeling we experience under optimal light and water conditions. It also gives evidence to the importance of maintaining a balance of the water in our bodies.

Timing – When to drink

Not all times are created equal – when it comes to drinking water, too. While listening to your own body is the best personalized strategy, some helpful general guidelines are these:

- Do not drink a lot of fluids (of any kind) before going to bed. Otherwise your sleep may be disturbed and not as restful.

- Do not drink extra fluids during or immediately after meal time. Instead, leave a gap of at least 30 minutes, or take in fluids before that meal. (Otherwise, your digestive system's work will be negatively impacted.)

- Start your day by replenishing fluids – e.g., drinking a glass of honey-laced warm water, perhaps with some lemon inside (if you like the taste). Note that if you are bringing the water to a boiling temperature, it is best to let it cool down first to reach body temperature before adding the honey.

- Drink a glass of (purified) water before taking a shower or a bath. (The above suggestion for replenishing fluids serves this purpose also.) This way your body's hydration needs will be more fully met, leading to less internal thirst for new fluid absorption through the skin. (The assumption here is that your available drinking water is of higher quality than the tap water which is fed to your shower head.)

- Your body may need more water and more frequently than usual (as previously mentioned) whenever you are cleansing / detoxing (physically, emotionally, mentally), doing a fast, nursing a baby, or have recently received energy healing.

Channels – How fluids enter your body

Just because you do not eat it or drink it does not mean it does not enter your body.

Fluids such as water enter your body most often through the mouth – when you consciously drink them. However, this is not the only pathway inward. The skin, as the largest organ in the human body, is another big gateway through which fluids enter (and leave) your body. So it is important to be conscious about not only what you drink directly, but more generally *what you expose your skin to*. Because of the skin's tendency to absorb what is on it, including any impurities, you are in fact giving tacit permission to everything you put on your skin to enter your system.

This includes tap water during showers / baths (which likely contains chlorine, fluoride, and other harmful chemicals, as discussed), and it also includes soap, lotion, anti-perspiration products, sunscreen, and other cosmetics. Many such so called personal care products are known to contain artificial preservatives, heavy metals (e.g., lead, cadmium, etc.), alcohols (e.g., propylene glycol), and a range of other harmful chemicals. [18.14]

Hence, you can limit your unconscious, back-channel exposure by:

- installing water filters on shower heads and faucets, or (even more effective) installing a water filtration device at the point of entry to your home; and

- consciously selecting personal care products by reading labels and staying informed on the health effects of common ingredients.

~

One small action step you can take today: Experiment with how much water is optimal for you by consuming half of your body weight in ounces every day. Try this for three days. Check in to see how you feel. Are there any changes in your appetite, cravings, or sleep? What does the color of your urine tell you? Do you need to increase or reduce your water intake?

Then, for the next three days drink to thirst. Pay attention to the same factors, and compare to your observations from the previous three days. Which method worked better for you in meeting your needs and improving how you feel?

Need an added challenge? For three days, jot down separately how many ounces of hydrating versus dehydrating fluids you consumed daily. At the end of each day, what was the individual tally for each category? What did you learn from the results? What did your urine color reveal this time?

Then, for the next four days commit to consuming only hydrating fluids, with no sugar added. Did you feel differently during and after this? If yes, in what ways? Are you noticing any shifts in food cravings and/or sleep patterns?

Part III:

Beyond Food – How Nutrition Relates to the Rest of Your Life

19: My body is giving me signals, but how do I learn to interpret them (easily)?

Curiously, some people take better care of their cars than they do of their bodies. They service their cars regularly, respond to low oil indications, stop at a gas station when the fuel gauge is fast approaching "Empty," etc. Yet they do not listen as keenly or respond to the indications their bodies give them. Perhaps they do not know how to interpret those signals.

Observe intently
Just as you listen to a friend keenly when they speak, you can also listen to your body when it "speaks" to you:

- How do you know when you are hungry? Your stomach growls.

- How do you know you are tired or sleepy? You feel heaviness and perhaps yawn.

- How do you know when you are stressed out? Your shoulders feel tense, you may be clenching your teeth, or may be more easily distracted in your thoughts.

These are some ways that your body "speaks" to you. [19.1] Signals, such as in the preceding examples are obvious and cannot be missed, hence are easy to connect and interpret. However, there are other signals that are equally powerful, yet more subtle. For example:

- You may suddenly crave sweets – possibly due to inadequate hydration.

- You may experience low energy after eating a particular food / meal – informing you that this particular food item (or a combination of items) is taking more time to break down and digest, leaving you feeling sapped and less energetic.

It is well known that your body speaks to you at all times. The question is, "Whenever your body speaks, are you paying attention, noticing, and interpreting properly?" And consequently, "Are you responding appropriately based on what you have understood?"

Below are some more examples of how your body may speak to you (perhaps daily). Are you aware of the possible meaning behind each case?

Type of body signals	Possible meanings
craving foods from your childhood	"missing home" or missing a specific person from your childhood (e.g., mom, dad, aunt, a friend), whom you associate with that food
a strong desire for a specific taste (sweet, salty, sour, pungent, bitter, astringent)	having eaten too much of the other tastes lately and very little of that presently desired taste – so your body is seeking to *balance* itself by "nudging" you to choose that "missing" taste, delivered (hopefully) via a wholesome food choice
often getting hungry soon after having eaten a meal	perhaps you did not chew your food well; or you ate too fast; or you ate mindlessly, in a mechanical fashion, not paying attention to what went in; or you were emotionally disturbed while eating; or your meal was nutritionally deficient; etc.
palpable emotional sensations in the company of certain people	stomach may cringe if there is a mismatch of your respective energies (e.g., peaceful vs. aggressive); heart would soar if you vibe well with a person, and the relationship is positive and uplifting to you
pain or discomfort in the groin or pelvic region	often associated with harboring envious thoughts. [19.2] Are you willing to let go of such thoughts and emotions, as the price to heal? [19.3]

Note the connection between certain signals manifesting physically, but having an interpretation in the emotional, mental, or non-physical realms.

How to connect within?
Just as you regularly check-in with your electronic devices for new

emails or messages, you can build-in a daily practice of checking-in with yourself by asking, "Dear body of mine, what message do you have for me today?" and listening for what you sense just after posing the question. With *regular practice* of listening keenly, you will learn to recognize where your body wants to direct your focus and attention. If you get into the habit of consistently tuning into your body, you will find that it becomes easier and easier to correctly interpret its signals and messages to you. The value of the communication you receive will be more than worth the effort of the practice that it takes to develop the skill of listening intently and interpreting signals.

How do you develop your abilities to tune in and listen to your body's signals? A number of paths can help you in that regard so long as you *practice consistently* whichever you choose. Some examples include: daily meditation, yoga, a peaceful and non-competitive form of martial arts (e.g., Aikido), muscle testing[42], or even taking conscious deep breaths.

It is recommended that you devote at least 30 minutes each day for many practices like those. However, even if you could only take 5 to 10 minutes, ideally twice a day, it would serve you well to start developing body awareness, which over time will enhance your ability to hear messages from your body. In essence, any practice that *slows you down enough* to be able to be mindful and conscious of what is unfolding within and around you, will help to expand your awareness. Even in a serious time crunch, you can still benefit by taking three conscious, deep breaths – directing your focus and awareness in those few moments toward your inhalations and exhalations. This serves to slow you down just a bit, creating a small degree of spaciousness within.

Benefits of understanding your body's signals

The above practices – including physical activities, exercises, sports, yoga, meditation, and games that you truly enjoy – are known to rewire the brain, bringing about positive effects, including development of self-awareness. [19.4, 19.5, 19.6]

---

[42] For more information on muscle testing, visit §2 and the References section.

Being able to interpret your body's signals has other benefits, too. It empowers you to serve your needs more effectively, offering your body and mind what they truly need (rather than what they may superficially want). It also helps to improve your confidence in being able to do so consciously. This in turn allows you to develop a non-adversarial relationship with yourself – with no guilt, no self-repression, and greater acceptance and self-care.

~

One small action step you can take today: The next time you experience a craving, instead of indulging immediately, take three slow and deep conscious breaths. Then ask yourself, "Dear body of mine, do you truly desire [state the craving] now or is it something else?" Take a few seconds to keenly listen for responses in the form of a feeling or a sensation. Try this experiment of checking within every time you experience a craving for the following three days. What was your body trying to tell you? What was different, if any, about this experience of tuning within? What did you learn about your relationship to cravings?

Need an added challenge? Commit to one form of mindfulness practice, such as yoga, meditation, a martial art form, tai chi, qigong, or a nature hike. Practice it for at least 30 minutes every day for a week. (Alternatively, you may choose to practice for at least 15 minutes twice a day, if that is easier for you.) How do you feel at the end of the week? Describe your sensations. Were you able to observe any shifts in your approach to routine tasks you do, and to habitual responses you have to stimuli in your world? Are you able to listen to your bodily signals better than you used to? How may you further fine-tune your capacity to listen to your physical, mental, and emotional needs? Are you open to consistently implementing some of these practices in your life (perhaps even ones you have not yet given a try) to improve your awareness?

20: I know what foods are good for my body, but why do I keep choosing ones that hurt me?

The power of habit

You already know that some foods are better for you than others, don't you? Yet, sometimes you find yourself choosing foods that are not as good for you – or even harmful for you in the long run. Why does this discrepancy happen? We are all creatures of habit. We have been brought up with specific habits and ideas, including those related to food, eating, and nourishment. We rarely, if ever, question these habits – unless specifically challenged (by a person or by a painful life experience) to do so. As long as those ideas that were passed on to us are nurturing and uplifting, all is well. Otherwise, our habitual "autopilot" choices hurt us slowly but surely.

Some common "habitual" traps that we often find ourselves in are the result of our beliefs. For example, we may believe that others have dominion over us and hence shift the responsibility onto them thinking, "*That's how I grew up and that's what people around me did.*" We may also use other excuses like, "*I just can't help it. It tastes so good,*" or lack self-discipline and think, "*Oh, just this one time won't hurt,*" or "*Okay, I'll do it some day, but not right now.*"

To make a change in habits, *awareness* and *self-discipline* are needed. Such a change is indeed possible to accomplish, with persistence, typically within a few weeks. It involves releasing the old and building new sustaining habits that honor you.

"Engineered" taste

Making things more challenging for you, in our modern society tastes are routinely "engineered" in order to be made more appealing – indeed, addictive – to the consumer. Sweet and salty tastes are often artificially recreated in a lab. Humans have been genetically predisposed (through evolutionary adaptation over the millennia) to associate sweet tastes with the desirable presence of energy-rich nutrients. Modern-day food marketers have been taking advantage of this inborn trait – creating processed foods, "spiked" with re-engineered sweet tastes, and using harmful chemicals. Their goal has been to entice you to pick their food product, which now has a "built-in" messenger to your senses: that this food item is supposedly energy-rich in nutrients. Once your senses become tricked, you can grow addicted to this food by choosing it over and over again. [20.1]

Food manufacturers, food marketers, and "flavorists" have been working hand-in-hand to create more addicting foods, packaged attractively. [20.2] Would you expect foods that are not commonly considered sweets, to still be loaded with much sugar? They often are. Examples include white breads, breakfast cereals, yogurts, some varieties of ketchup, relishes, salad dressings, sauces, soups, and marinades. Just as sugar is sneaked into foods, salt too is often added to foods that you might otherwise not expect to see much of it. Examples are breakfast cereals, vegetable juices, canned vegetables, roasted nuts, ketchup, relishes, and many more. [20.3] Many restaurants too have designed the "perfect" addicting taste (e.g., Thai curries, sesame orange chicken, Alfredo sauce, etc.) by combining sugar and salt in proportions that are higher than what is generally recommended. Most processed food manufacturers add considerable amounts of salt per serving size in order to help preserve the freshness of the ingredients in their packaged foods. Salt is also commonly added to bring out other flavors in the products.

Therefore it becomes vitally important to learn to interpret nutrition labels on packaged foods, including serving sizes, in order to estimate how much sugar or salt is contained in the amounts that you normally eat. Such awareness will help you make wiser choices, in case you have been over-consuming such questionable foods. Once you are empowered with the relevant knowledge, you can consciously weigh your short-term pleasures (often delivered via addictive and nutritionally deficient foods) versus your long-term wellbeing and happiness (delivered via non-addictive and nutrient-dense foods).

If you blindly follow your senses, and your senses have already been tricked, your body is subconsciously "running on autopilot," so your ability to make conscious choices may be diminished. If you find yourself defaulting to, say, ice cream and cookies to satisfy each one of your desires for a sweet taste, consider *consciously* replacing most of these foods with sweet-tasting fruits and veggies. Observe your senses over time, and notice any shifts.

The good and the bad choices

Examples of nutrient-rich sweet and yummy foods are: cherries, blueberries, carrots, yams, and corn, among many others. [20.4] At the same time, consciously avoid fast, cheap, and convenience foods, including those found at fast food restaurants. Here is a brief list of some of the most popular – yet *very unhealthy* – foods carried by a majority of grocery and convenience stores' prepared food sections, as well as in fast food chains: soda, fried chicken, bacon cheeseburger, French fries, milk shake, pepperoni pizza, nachos, hotdogs, and many more! [20.5]

In the end, foods that only tickle your taste buds but offer little nutrient value will have negative consequences for you. So make the smarter choice in favor of foods that not only tickle your taste buds but are health promoting as well. It is certainly possible to choose *both healthy and tasty* foods. The options are plentiful, and the myth that you have to decide between one and the other is just that: a myth.

~

One small action step you can take today: For one day, choose to consume only foods that are flavored by Nature and not by "flavorists." Each time you pick up a food or a snack, ask yourself: "Is this a gift from Nature?" If you hear a 'yes', go ahead and enjoy the gift; if you are in doubt, set it aside. Tally how many times you picked Nature-made foods, and how many times it was the "engineered" foods. What can you discern from the numbers? Were there any surprising revelations? If yes, what were they? Which parts of this exercise were easy for you, and which were not so easy? In what other ways can you improve upon your habituated ways of choosing foods? Are you willing to extend this way of choosing your foods for another few days?

Need an added challenge? Scan your pantry and fridge. Make a pile of foods that are Nature-made, and another pile of foods that are (likely) created by food manufacturers and "flavorists." How many in each category did you find? Were you pleasantly surprised or shocked by the tally? For the next one week, commit to eating only

Nature-made foods, or foods created by conscious food manufacturers who use only Nature-made ingredients (i.e., with no added chemicals, artificial flavors, sugars, sugar-free substitutes, or salt). Did you notice any shifts in the way you felt – physically, mentally, or emotionally? If yes, how? If not, why do you think it is so? What other food choices and/or food companies can you identify that "fit the bill" of being healthy for you? Would you be willing to give them a try?

21: I have started making changes, but I encounter roadblocks. How do I keep going effectively?

The beginning of a change

As you may have observed from personal experience, as soon as you begin to adopt certain changes in your life and are well intentioned to make these become your new default, you often take a few steps backwards (instead of staying on course) into old ways of being and doing things. Why does this happen? There are several reasons. Just when you seem to be making progress, a tendency to sabotage your efforts can get in your way, as if to claim on your behalf, "*I don't deserve all this good,*" thereby bringing you back to your original set point [21.1]. Another reason relates to the concept of *homeostasis* – the innate tendency of the body to resist frequent changes. [21.2] Yet another reason can be associated with the "side effects" of making positive shifts: old toxins (physical and emotional) get released in the process, which could be painful (literally and figuratively), prompting you to pause your forward momentum, wondering if there is something wrong with what you have set out to do. As the saying goes, "*It often gets worse before it gets better.*" In that same light, it is important to realize that when you start cleaning up your diet (or any other aspect of your life), you will gradually release an old, deeply buried build-up of stale and toxic substances and emotions. These must be released and cleansed out of your system before new, positive changes can take hold and become your second nature. Therefore, by staying the course and not giving up you will meet a healthier version of yourself, in time. As you start making better food choices, your head will clear up gradually, your brain will not feel foggy any more, and you will naturally begin to take better care of yourself – starting to prefer foods that are better suited for you.

Be patient with your body

Do you find yourself saying, "*I've tried to make a change, but didn't see a difference in the result*" or "*It's too hard to change*"? Remember that change can take time. You probably did not "see a difference," because you either did not implement the change correctly (e.g., choosing to eliminate gluten, but inadvertently consuming it as croutons on your salad) or did so intermittently rather than regularly (e.g., saying you will eliminate gluten for 21 days, but eating it once every 2 days). In the above examples, although you were well intentioned about the change, you experienced backslides as your body did not get the chance to get accustomed to the new state of being. Allow yourself sufficient time to get used to any changes you are incorporating in your life. You did not arrive overnight at your present condition (from which you are seeking relief), so now that you have chosen to make that U-turn towards vibrant health, it also may not happen overnight. Do not think about it being "too hard" to change – just focus on making small and regular steps forward in the direction of your intent. It will serve you well to be patient with yourself and let your body adjust accordingly. You may also affirm,

"This is a false idea I have bought into. It is safe to change it. I am open and willing to make a change. I have the power to change it. So be it. And so it is."

All eyes on me?

If you are one who has a special health condition (e.g., a severe allergy or food sensitivity) or who has made a conscious commitment to eat healthfully, then you may have experienced mental roadblocks such as: *"I don't want to stand out as the one who rejects food options in a company of friends,"* or *"I have a special health condition, which makes me uncomfortable to go out with friends,"* or *"I do not want friends to be inconvenienced about treating me differently due to my health situation,"* and so on. Just know that it is alright – and indeed recommended – that you be your own advocate, as who else can advocate for you better than yourself? As you become increasingly more comfortable in your own skin, standing up for yourself with a willingness to receive what honors your needs, you also allow others to respect your health needs when you are in their company. Then you will also become a voice and an inspiration for those who find themselves in a similar predicament. Best of all, you will enjoy spending time in the company of friends, and sharing a dining experience with them without the burden of self-imposed roadblocks.

Sustaining changes in practice

Although sustaining positive changes may seem like a journey you are taking alone, in practice *it takes a team* to help sustain positive changes. *Who and what you surround yourself with* – the people as well as the environment – will to a large extent determine the results you experience. If you have people who hold you accountable while supporting you with the changes you are embarking upon, it will help you greatly in continuing your forward momentum. If you have often said to yourself, *"It's hard to make changes,"* then a team of clear-headed witnesses and passionate cheerleaders, honest advisors and benevolent critics can ease your journey. The human tendency for self-sabotage and the natural feeling of discomfort during the cleansing of toxic releases make it crucial to have such qualified mentors and a support system. This is especially true when slip-ups happen or, better yet, before they happen – to anticipate potential roadblocks that may hinder your desired changes. Don't forget to notice and celebrate even the smallest positive changes along the way (e.g., if you have started taking one conscious breath before meals). This will help you to stay motivated and on track.

Close family members may be well meaning, yet when it comes to making shifts, they are often among the first naysayers and doubters (e.g., telling you why you should not be doing this), or pretending sages (e.g., who know "better" alternatives for you). This can create an environment not conducive to successfully making changes. While it is useful to be open to suggestions (for people may have nuggets to share), you would be best served by remaining in control of your life's choices – for who else knows what is best for your body, mind, and soul than you yourself! Many of us have a tendency to wait for others in the family to come on board with our "new idea" related to healthier choices. It is recommended that as soon as you realize the value of making a shift for yourself, you begin implementing the changes, and do so without making big upfront announcements. Once you start experiencing positive health benefits, it will be even more compelling and authentic for you, and it would be hard for family members to ignore or argue against the results. Moreover, you can become an inspiration for them to join in on the journey, or at least this can be an impetus for them to reclaim their own health and on their own terms. It is not necessary to wait for others to catch up with you or to validate your choices and ideas before you begin implementing those.

Deeper issues
Do you notice repeated negative thought patterns around your body image or self-judgment that have made it difficult for you to make positive shifts in your life? Are you feeling stuck and unable to move forward? Do you often speak in self-demeaning ways before others?

If you have already used the tools described in this book, and yet still find yourself unable to make progress, it may be that the challenges you are facing require a more in-depth healing, perhaps not only on a physical level. To offer you the proper support on your healing journey, we suggest that you seek out a team of qualified healers, doctors, coaches, and/or therapists.

~

One small action step you can take today: Pick one food item that you know does *not* serve your best health interest, yet one that you nonetheless consume daily. For three days do not eat that particular food item. Notice your physical sensations. How is your body reacting? Is the change easy or hard on your body? How was your mood on day 1, on day 2, and at the end of day 3? Were you feeling better or worse with each passing day? Why do you think this is so? Are you willing to stay the course, and allow the change to become a habit?

Need an added challenge? Identify a health goal that you have been contemplating for a while but have not yet implemented due to peer pressure or possible naysayers in the family. This week, give yourself permission to go ahead despite any doubts. Share your goal with family members or friends, and see how they respond. Is your resolve strengthened or weakened as a result? Will you still move forward in the face of "opposition" or lack of support? If you are still harboring doubts, what specific steps could you take to help you move forward with strong conviction?

22: How do I make good choices when I am at a party or any social setting?

When you regularly and consciously eat healthy, nutritious foods, an invitation to a party or social gathering may seem a bit daunting given the likelihood that available food choices may not be as health affirming as your normal "diet." Still, there are ways to help alleviate this concern and still join the party. Here are a few tested practices:

- Eat a healthy meal or snack 30 minutes to an hour before the event, so you would not be ravenously hungry at the start of the party. Include healthy sweet and crunchy foods such as carrots, cherries, banana, kale, etc., so that you do not crave those textures and/or tastes (via unhealthy foods like chips and cookies) as much at the party.

- Etiquette permitting, consider taking nutritious food to share with others at the party, perhaps offering it as a gift to the host for inviting you. Think "nutritious food" in lieu of (or in addition to) flowers or a box of chocolates! Bringing food to share may not always be an option; do the best you can, given the circumstances.

- Fill up at least 80% of your plate with "whole" foods such as fruits, veggies, and/or minimally processed foods with fewer ingredients. Then you will have little room left for "not so nutritious" options such as cake, ice cream, chips, juice, etc.

- Shift your vibration (state of mind) from one of apprehension to one of openness and receptivity by blessing the food and mentally stating an intention of how you wish it to be in your body. For example, *"Thank you to all the plants and animals who have generously contributed to this blessed, nutritious, delicious, healthful, and clean food. May only the highest vibrations from this food flow through me."* Also, while getting ready for the party, remind yourself and affirm (silently or out loud) a message of self-empowerment, e.g., *"I am the master of my body, and I only choose foods that nourish it,"* or *"I am empowered to make conscious food choices."* Feel free to experiment with the choice of words, and coin your own positive affirmations[43] that resonate with you, putting you in a state of gratitude and empowerment.

- Some of us have been taught to not waste food. Still, remember that in the spirit of not wasting food, do not consume food that is wasting *you* – you are *not a trash bin*! For example, if you are handed pre-plated foods and you prefer to not eat some of it, you can honor your guidance by removing those parts and eating what is agreeable to you.

- Set an example by inviting friends and offering food that is delicious, nutritious, healthy, and celebratory. Who said that party food cannot be a combination of magnificent qualities!

~

One small action step you can take today: At the start of every meal, for a period of 3 days, take about 10 seconds to slow down and express a silent "thank you" (you may use the affirmation of gratitude mentioned above, if you wish) to all the resources that have gone into the creation of the meal laid out before you. Did you notice, over time, any shifts in the way you related to your food? What felt different about your mealtime experience? How was your mood at the start, during, and at the end of each meal?

Need an added challenge? The next time you are invited to a party or a social gathering (especially events where "not so nutritious" food items are likely to be served), eat a healthy meal or snack shortly before the event. If possible, include a variety of different tastes, as well as some protein and fiber to keep you satiated. (If you need some ideas, please refer to the Appendices.) Notice if the foods you pick at the gathering are different now. How was your appetite at the party? Were your choices a big departure from your norm at gatherings? If yes, how; if not, what may have influenced your choices (e.g., discomfort about being different, fear of embarrassment, etc.)? If you found this experiment helpful, are you open to incorporating it regularly in similar future situations?

---

[43] An affirmation is a statement made in the first person, in present tense, setting an intention. It is important to carefully choose the words in it, since words have power to create your future.

23: What other factors might influence my food choices?

So far we have discussed the value of making conscious food choices. What if your choices are impacted also by circumstances beyond your conscious control?

External influencers
The days when you choose to (or must) eat out, be it at your workplace or school, in restaurants, at social gatherings or events, you likely have far fewer choices of a "healthier" kind. This ties in with the earlier discussion about who drives the choices you make around food. Is it you, your family, your friends, your workplace or school, or food marketing companies (offering you the lure of easy, "convenience" foods)? This is something to observe and think through carefully.

Beliefs around food
Every household has its philosophy around food; something that is often passed down from generation to generation, perhaps even subconsciously. What is your family's "story" around food, eating, health, and wellbeing? What have you grown up hearing and observing? Some commonly repeated ideas include:

- *"Home food is the best food on Earth."*

- *"Eating healthy is hard to do."*

- *"Eat less to stay well."*

- *"Eat more to become strong."*

- *"Eat more so you don't get hungry soon."*

- *"I get fat even if I simply look at food."*

- *"Eat it all – for the sake of people who can only afford very little."*

- *"Eat it no matter what; we don't throw away food in this home."*

- *"Don't play with your food, it is sacred and meant to be eaten."*

Do you recognize any of these? Is your family's idea a version of some of them? Such ideas and stories greatly shape your relationship to all aspects of food, and consequently affect your decisions around what you eat, when you eat, how much you eat, and why you eat. So it is important to realize that these ideas are simply *beliefs* that do not necessarily represent truth.

Practical tips for improving food-related choices
Here are some helpful daily practices:

- *Eating slowly and mindfully* and *chewing food properly* will enable you to easily decipher when your stomach is full, thereby helping you to derive maximum benefit from the nutrients you consume. This will also help to consciously control your portion size as well as the types of foods you pick.

- A *silent affirmation of gratitude for the meal* that is laid out before you will intentionally slow you down and delay the instant gratification from the first bite you might otherwise quickly gulp down. Slowing down at the start would help you connect with your food better. Just as you greet a friend at your doorstep first before you two sit down to tea, you can also "receive" or "greet" your food first before digging right into it. In general, slowing down while eating will also help you to digest better.

In addition, you can positively influence your food choices via some non-food related practices:

- *Regularly perform physical activities that you find enjoyable.* When you truly enjoy an activity, your body releases "happy" neurotransmitters (e.g., endorphins) that elevate your mood, help you relax, and improve your presence of mind. All this allows you to make better choices (including around food).

- *A consistent, restorative nighttime sleep* helps to regulate a healthy appetite the following day. Cravings are minimized, energy levels are improved, mood is brightened, and as a result you make wiser choices.

~

One small action step you can take today: For one day, whenever you eat a meal or a snack, make it a point to chew each bite between 20 and 40 times (depending upon how soft or hard the food items are) for at least the first seven mouthfuls. Does your food taste differently as a result? How does it feel to consciously slow down your pace of eating, by measured chewing? Did you consume less or more food at each meal? Why might that be?

Need an added challenge? Identify your family's "stories" around food, nutrition, and health. In a journal, list the various ways that these stories influence your present relationship with these aspects of wellbeing, including what you eat, when you eat, how much you eat, and why you eat. Notice and reflect on how an improved clarity on this subject shifts your approach to your wellbeing. If a "story" is a supportive one, would you continue "living it"? If not, are you open to write a new, empowering "story" in its place?

24: If I had little spare time and wished to make one change to my nutrition / lifestyle to begin with, what would be most beneficial to do?

In every moment, you can decide which change is most beneficial *for you* by staying focused on the following *strategies* (describing *what* you can do and *why* you want to do it) along with a few related *"tactics"* (describing *how* specifically you can do it).

Strategies (the "what" and "why")

- **Consider your own unique context**
  Apply the knowledge and awareness you have already developed of the main principles of sound nutrition in the context of *your unique body type* and *your unique life situation*. While a general recommendation can be good, a personalized suggestion can work even better for you. It honors your specific needs and potential constraints (including how much time you are willing to devote regularly to making the change you desire, how supportive your environment is, etc.).

- **Choose changes that energize you**
  Changes are most sustainable when they feel motivating and the result is energizing to you. To find out what those desirable changes are, ask yourself:

  - "What feels most nourishing to me as a human being?" and

  - "Which foods give my body both energy and satisfaction?"

  Over the course of a few days, take your time to experiment with possible answers. Keenly observe how you feel. If you feel more vibrant, make those nourishing, energizing, and satisfying choices a staple of your life. Still, your answers to the above questions may evolve over time. That is quite normal – you will be honoring your specific context and new life situation yet again.

- **Minimize the natural stress from going through changes**
  Stress can have a negative effect on your motivation and

commitment to changes. So it is best to take proactive steps to consciously minimize stress. The "80-20 rule" we suggest below is one tactic that can help to minimize stress in practice.

Tactics (the "how")

- **If you are on the go...**
  Identify your ideal meal combinations, as well as ideal snacks, separately. Keep healthy snacks prepackaged (one serving size each) and handy wherever you spend most of your time. This is useful when hunger strikes and you feel the urge to have something to eat. You may keep snacks in your bag, in your car, and at your workplace.

  This approach has numerous benefits. It eliminates the compulsion to visit a fast food chain, it gives you what you consciously chose as the best snack for you, it saves you time, and it saves you money too. [24.1, 24.2]

- **Make meal preparation be a pleasant and shared experience**
  Invite your family and/or friends who have a similar outlook on healthy living to engage with you regularly and share in the creation of healthy meals. This will save you time, and will provide an uplifting experience of emotional support to all participants. Some fun ideas to consider are:

  o cooking together;

  o preparing vegetables and herbs ahead of time and in bulk for an entire week;

  o sharing the prepared ingredients with the people who help you in your efforts;

  o offering a meal to your "willing kitchen helpers" in exchange for their assistance;

  o turning this into a "work party" experience – with food, music, and merrymaking, while chopping, packing, and stacking away!

- **Follow an "80-20 rule" for maintaining a balance**
  The idea is this: you commit to getting the best nutrition you know of (i.e., meals that are healthy, nutritious, and true to your individual constitution) *at least 80% of the time*. However, you also build-in a "flaw allowance" that offers you some leeway – permitting you to not be as strict and "pristine" for the remaining 20% of the time. So if you did veer off course occasionally due to circumstances forcing you to leave your perfect trajectory, you would not feel guilty or judge yourself for having had a slip-up. You are still being authentic and honoring of yourself.

  For example, if a child at a birthday party wants to partake in tasting the cake, it is prudent health-wise to remove artificial colorings, take a small-size piece, check its sweetness (to avoid eating much sugar), bless the food, then enjoy it with no regrets. Or if you have a cookie each day while otherwise eating healthy, nutrition-packed meals, you will likely be fine. Similarly, if you eat organic foods daily, but are offered a slice of conventional pizza at a friend's place or a non-organic meal on an occasion, it may not have as much of an adverse impact on your health.

  This "80-20 rule" may relieve you from the burden of always maintaining a "perfect eater" status, which can be a source of significant stress, especially in situations when the best food options are not readily available.

  To sustain good health, however, it is important to *apply this rule with care and discernment* – only opting for alternatives (including "treats") that are made with real ingredients, not artificial flavors and/or additives. The reason is that *regular* indulgences of so called "food-like substances" or foods that you may be unknowingly sensitive to can cause a great deal of harm to your body.

  Once you are riding high on the above "80-20 rule" and are comfortable complying with it, you may challenge yourself to a higher "90-10 rule"!

~

One small action step you can take today: Prepackage six individual single-serving, nutrition-rich snacks. Place a couple of each in various locations besides your home (e.g., in your car, cubicle at work or school, backpack, handbag, etc.). The next time you get hungry and there is no easy access to nutritious food, you may reach for one of the snack packs and enjoy it with gratitude in your heart. How long did these prepackaged snacks last until you had to put together more of them? What did you most like or not like about this process? What else could you do so that when you are on-the-go, your food choices would work for you, instead of against you?

Need an added challenge? Throw a potluck or tea party at home and invite 2-3 friends, who could also use some help in prepping their veggies and/or pre-cooking some food items (so that their weekday meals become easier to put together). What was your most valuable take-away from sharing a couple of hours with like-minded people and supporting one another in your quest for a more healthful lifestyle? How did your friends feel about this experience? Are you inspired to implement this idea periodically? What other ideas come to mind as you contemplate creating easy-to-prepare, healthy, home-cooked meals each day?

25: How can children be empowered to make sound nutrition choices by themselves?

Creating an empowering movement
The skills you learn and practice in life take a *larger meaning* when you are able to pass them on to others and empower them to make positive changes for themselves too. It creates a movement, whereas before that it was just about you and your choices. Every movement starts slow, with a handful of friends and family. Children can be especially eager and open to adopt (new) practices – they do not (yet) have the self-imposed restrictions that many adults have – if your approach to empowering them is right. But first it is important to take the baby steps to empower yourself, since *"you cannot give to another what you do not already have inside of you."*

Becoming the change you wish to see
Young ones often model after grown-ups' actions, don't they? To be a positive role model for them, manage yourself well along this journey of self-care and healthy eating. Backslides may occur every now and then, but as you train yourself to be aware of slip-ups (with the right focus and intention), you will be able to take the "lessons" from such experiences, and recalibrate your habits. Maintaining a healthy lifestyle is a continual process of incremental adjustments, rather than a rigid "success or failure" proposition. The journey to wellbeing (and healthy eating, as part of it) is not an all-or-nothing experience, but *a process of re-centering time and again* whenever a shift in an unusual direction occurs or when your individual constitution or context change. You will then be able to more easily pivot in a direction that serves your highest health and wellness goals.

Doing all this *consciously and consistently* will send a powerful message to a child who observes you.

This process can be better understood with an example. You (and/or your child) may have set an intention to chew your food slowly and mindfully at each meal, after you have learned about the health benefits of doing so. But for some reason you do so for only one of your daily meals. Instead of labeling yourself a "failure" or someone who cannot keep commitments, simply notice the slip-up and pick yourself back up during your next mealtime opportunity. If you find yourself in a rush during all of your mealtimes, revisit your original intention and recalibrate the commitment to reflect your deeper aspirations. Take into account your daily duties, and make sure they are compatible with your recalibrated commitment.

For example, you may reduce from three to one the number of daily mealtimes when you resolve to chew slowly and properly. Later, as you regain your footing with comfort, you may gradually build upon your small "success." You are more likely to experience a lasting positive shift when you make changes incrementally. In this case, a consistent "proper chewing" during at least one of your daily mealtimes is likely to induce a good feeling overall – physically, emotionally, and mentally (due to better digestion resulting in greater energy and enhanced mental clarity). Building on that, you may then become inspired to do the same even more often, perhaps at all mealtimes (and at snack time too). This approach of *making incremental shifts by noting (your own body's) feedback and recalibrating* based on that (while being gentle with yourself all the while) will help you and your child to sustain changes you make over a lifetime.

Helping to deconstruct cravings
The above idea connects well with the practical steps for cultivating body awareness and tuning within, which we explored in some detail previously. Children can be empowered with such practical tools to be able to decipher the signals that their bodies give them. One caveat is that there may be a tendency for children – as they take their first steps practicing the process of tuning-in – to occasionally misinterpret any cravings to mean a cue that must be satisfied. For example, a child may say that her body desires something sweet. How can you tell for sure that this signal is genuine and not a physiological (e.g., dehydration / thirst) or emotional (e.g., feeling bored or lonely) "gap" that needs to be addressed instead? It takes practice. The more consistently you apply the practical steps (mentioned in §2) to cultivate body awareness, the better you will become at interpreting your own bodily signals and discerning whether you are experiencing a craving or a genuine desire for a certain type of food. Once you, the parent or caretaker, become one who is empowered, you could support a child by helping her

deconstruct her bodily signals by regularly checking in and jointly discovering any patterns underneath the craving.

Nurturing positive attitudes toward health and eating

Children behave like sponges. They absorb the energy or vibe of the predominant thoughts and ideas entertained or spoken by family members and others. It is therefore critical to pay close attention to your words, actions, and even non-verbal expressions related to the subject of food, health, and nutrition (or to any subject, for that matter). A positive spin on such ideas is fundamental. Otherwise a child may grow up with skewed notions around what it means to be optimally nourished and healthy, potentially leading to eating disorders, poor body image, and other similar avoidable conditions. What conversations take place in your household regarding food, eating, and health?

Actively engaging with family and community

Some positive ways to relate to one another around the subject of health and nutrition is to involve each member of the household to be actively engaged in some aspects of food preparation, including meal planning, purchasing ingredients, preparing, cooking, and cleaning up. Often taking children to visit a local farm to see how food is grown sustainably, and giving them the opportunity to pick some fruits and vegetables to take home, is a way to bring them genuinely close to the source of their food. They will begin to appreciate the effort it takes to cultivate healthy, seasonal produce, and will likely be open to eating it. Starting a small vegetable garden at home, where children participate actively, is also a fun way to keep them engaged. A visit to a Farmers' Market is another wonderful opportunity to see how many growers have collaborated to produce our food. Children can be empowered to make choices of fruits and vegetables they would like to buy that day in planning for the next meal.

$\sim$

One small action step you can take today: Pick a day and empower your child to plan all three family meals for that day. Encourage them to create a healthy and balanced meal for breakfast, lunch, and dinner. Enjoy preparing, cooking, and eating together as a family. What felt different about this particular day's mealtime experiences? Were you surprised at the child's ideas for meals? What did you learn about your child from this experience? How well did the child's choices reflect your own beliefs and behaviors around food and eating? What other ideas could you employ to inspire them to joyfully continue to make healthy food choices?

Need an added challenge? Make a trip with your child to a local organic / sustainable farm or to a Farmers' Market. Encourage your child to ask the farmer what inspires him/her to get up each day and work on the farm. Learn first-hand with your child about the farmer's opportunities and challenges in creating this bounty for us to enjoy. If farms or Farmers' Markets are not easily accessible where you live, then visit a local grocery store and encourage your child to inquire where the store gets the produce and how it gets delivered to the store. Let your child pick at least one bagful of fresh produce from your visit, and let him/her help you prepare a healthy meal. How did you and your child enjoy your visit and conversation with the farmer (or grocer)? What was something new that you and/or your child learned about the farmers and the farming practices (or about the source of produce in the grocery store)? How did your meal taste, now that you have an idea of where the food you prepared came from? What was different about this experience where you consciously involved your child to be an active participant?

26: Where can I find additional truthful information on these and similar topics? How do I tell the credibility of information I come across?

There are several websites, books, and documentaries where you can find additional reliable information on the topics we have touched upon in the questions above. We suggest that you cross-reference multiple sources when learning more about specific new topics. Here are some resources for your benefit:

General resources – nutrition, food industry, alternative therapies, holistic health, etc.
www.Mercola.com
www.GreenMedInfo.com
www.MichaelPollan.com
www.DrHyman.com
www.DrWeil.com
www.FoodBabe.com
www.TheDr.com
www.CureJoy.com

GMO resources
www.ResponsibleTechnology.org
www.VandanaShiva.com

Ayurveda resources
www.LifeSpa.com
www.AyurvedaSeattle.com

Books
"Why We Get Fat", by Gary Taubes
"The Real Truth about Sugar", by Dr. Robert Lustig
"Mind over Meds", by Dr. Andrew Weil
"Integrative Nutrition", by Joshua Rosenthal
"The Omnivore's Dilemma", by Michael Pollan
"Eat Fat, Get Thin", by Dr. Mark Hyman
"Food Body", by Sadhguru

Videos & Documentaries

"Fed-up"

"Supersize me"

"Fat, sick & nearly dead"

"Genetic roulette"

"Food matters"

"Food, Inc."

"The human experiment"

"Yuck – a 4th grader's short documentary about school lunch"

"Nutrition detectives"

"Cooked"

"Consumed"

The above listing reflects only a small fraction of the sources of truthful information on the subjects of food, health, nutrition, sustainable living, and beyond.

In order to ensure that your source of information is reliable, check to see if the research data / information, scientific study, meta-analysis, or any other type of study – as the case may be – is being done by individuals or institutions, including government agencies, that:

(a) have no vested interest in a specific outcome of the subject of research / study;

(b) have not received – in part or whole – monetary funds from organizations (e.g., chemical companies, large bio-techs, agri-businesses, pharmaceutical industries, etc.) that have a vested interest in a specific outcome of the research / study.

If you come across other reliable resources, add them in appropriate categories to your expanding list.

~

One small action step you can take today: Pick one topic that is of interest to you from the information that you have so far taken in from the handbook. Take some time to research more on this topic. Select from one or more of the above mentioned resources or find your own reliable source. What new ideas did you learn from your research? How might you apply this knowledge in your own life?

Need an added challenge? Select a documentary film from the above suggested list to watch with family and/or friends. Take notes, if you prefer, while watching so as to remember salient features, suggestions, resources, and key people that are mentioned in the documentary. Once you finish watching, discuss amongst yourselves one change in each of your lives that the film inspired you to make. What immediate steps are you prepared to take toward implementing the desired change in your life? Go ahead, take those steps, and implement the change. We wish you well on your journey!

Conclusion

It is our sincere hope that the concepts discussed in this handbook are encouraging you to shift from the mindset of being solely a consumer of information to becoming an owner and implementer of ideas – an inspiration to others.

On this journey to achieving and maintaining optimum health, it will serve you well to remember that you are a *unique individual*, so a diet that is good for another may not necessarily be appropriate for you, and vice versa. (After all, there are 7 billion people on our planet, so there may well be 7 billion diets, too – including factors of food choice, portion size, methods of preparation, and so on.) Taking the time to assess your specific constitution, body type, and activity level (among other factors) is essential to choosing proper foods to help you maintain optimum health and vibrancy. Taking control of your nutrition choices in this manner is highly empowering – you no longer need to listen to and follow the latest "diet" fads out there, but rather be comfortable in the knowing, through your own *personal experience*, that your body feels well-nourished with foods that are not only delectable but are also easy to digest and absorb. Personalized and *consciously made nutrition choices* empower you, whereas copying what others are blindly adopting (e.g., following some diet research that appears "compelling") can often make you feel like a "victim of circumstance": if the "new diet" fails to deliver on its promise in your case, you might even stoop to blaming the "diet" or another individual for your lack of good health.

You always *do* have a choice, and the question is this: *Whose choice will you follow – yours or another's?*

Another key piece to self-empowerment is *self-awareness*. Tuning into your body and doing an honest assessment of how you are feeling is a powerful approach that can be applied in all areas of your life – not limited to your physical body. Particularly as this discussion refers to food, nutrition, and health, such an assessment will inform your food choices and what true nourishment means for you. Applying some of the tools discussed here, you will be able to learn how to better *decipher what your body tries to tell you.* Some of these tools enable you to slow down or pause for just long enough to be able to tune in and consciously listen to (rather than being oblivious to) the cues and signals of your body.

As the discussion has made evident, no matter what food choices you identify as your "ideal" diet, there are certain ingredients that most people acknowledge as being harmful to the human body (e.g., food additives, artificial colors and flavors, genetically modified foods, etc.). Likewise, there are many foods that receive universal kudos (e.g., many vegetables and fruits). Therefore, strive to incorporate in your daily diet plenty of fresh (and organic, when possible) vegetables and fruits. Whether you are vegan, paleo, pescatarian, omnivore, or have any other food preferences, you will benefit from eating generous servings of seasonal vegetables and fruits.

The food you eat "becomes you," helping build your cells, tissues, and organs, which in turn produce the right hormones and neurotransmitters, which in turn impact your mood and the way you think and focus. An understanding of yourself as an individual who nourishes not only the physical body with nutritious foods but, as a natural consequence, also the non-physical aspects (e.g., moods, emotions, intellect, etc.), will enable you to more fully grasp – and be in *conscious control* over – your motivations behind the everyday (food) choices you make. Food is indeed information!

What we offer throughout are *perspectives to consider, rather than prescriptions to follow.* There is nothing dogmatic or rigid about the nutrition- and health-related principles we share. Indeed, their timeless quality gives a lasting long-term value to the material. Still, you are invited to always check-in with yourself about *what is true for you* at any given moment.

Learning and adopting good nutrition habits requires sound knowledge on the one hand, and an open mind on the other. Teaching someone how to drive better immediately after they have had a collision may be hard to do – they may not be in a receptive state of mind yet. Similarly, teaching good nutrition habits to someone soon after they have fallen sick may be harder than expected – they may be overwhelmed by their ill health at that moment. Recovering from damages is possible, but harder. Instead, using *preventative care* and learning how to avoid trouble is fundamental to achieving and maintaining robust health.

In retrospect, it may seem that the human society's progression over time from hunter gatherer to agrarian to industrial revolution to chemical and genetic engineering is also one cause for the progressive degeneration of life on Earth as we know it. However, one constant here is the power and potential of human beings (i.e., us) who can embrace the "latest and greatest" tools and integrate them wisely with an intention of creating a sustainable choice for today and for generations to come. Instead of blaming evolution as has occurred over millennia, how about taking the responsibility to evolve ourselves consciously?

In this modern age when many people wish to be "ahead of the crowd," consider getting ahead also in health and wellbeing. Make conscious choices that honor your body, mind, and spirit. *Be the change* first among your family members and fellow human beings. This will start a ripple effect and inspire others to follow in your positive and practical footsteps.

May you grow to be a continued inspiration to all whose lives you touch!

Appendix A: Healthy "Sweet Treat" Alternatives

✓ Fresh whole fruits

✓ Dried fruits (with no added sugar)

✓ Raw nuts

✓ Apple or banana with nut butters

✓ Medjool dates stuffed with pecans, walnuts, or nut butter

✓ Porridge sweetened with a drizzle of maple syrup, raw honey or dried fruits

✓ Whole grain breads sweetened with dates, raisins, or bananas

✓ Unsweetened Greek yogurt with lightly sweetened granola / muesli or with a drizzle of raw honey

✓ Fruits (e.g., strawberries, banana, pineapple, etc.) dipped in melted dark chocolate

✓ Dark or raw chocolate

✓ Smoothies made with vegetables and fruits

✓ Freshly squeezed fruit juice (about 4-8oz serving per day)

✓ Homemade trail mixes with raw nuts and no-sugar added dried fruits (optional: add carob, dark chocolate chips, or cocoa nibs)

✓ Roasted sweet vegetables (e.g., carrots, yams, sweet potatoes, squashes, beets, parsnips, etc.) with a sprinkle of cinnamon powder or pumpkin pie spice mix (optional: add grass-fed butter or ghee) to resemble "fries"

✓ Dips made with sweet tasting vegetables (e.g., carrots, yams, sweet potatoes, squashes, beets, parsnips, etc.) and seasoned with spices of your choice

✓ Homemade popcorn with a light sprinkling of coconut sugar or date sugar

✓ Desserts (truffles, bars, puddings, etc.) made with dates, nuts, coconut flakes, non-dairy milk, and/or with natural, unrefined sweeteners such as maple syrup, coconut sugar, etc.)

✓ Baked or lightly grilled fruit (e.g., apple, pear, pineapple) with a dollop of unsweetened vanilla whipped cream

Note: We recommend using organic sources whenever possible – to avoid harmful pesticides, herbicides, and genetically engineered ingredients.

Appendix B: Healthy & Rich Sources of Protein

Vegetarian sources (preferably organic)

- ✓ Nuts – almonds, cashews, pistachios, walnuts, peanuts, hazelnuts, pine nuts, chestnuts, macadamias, pecans

- ✓ Seeds – pumpkin, chia, sunflower, hemp, sesame, flax

- ✓ Greek yogurt (unsweetened)

- ✓ Cottage cheese

- ✓ Beans – navy, pinto, black, garbanzo, kidney, mung

- ✓ Green vegetables – kale, collard, spinach, broccoli, asparagus, peas, edamame

- ✓ Bee pollen

- ✓ Royal jelly[44]

Non-vegetarian sources

- ✓ Organic and/or pastured eggs

- ✓ Wild-caught and/or sustainably raised smaller fish

- ✓ Organic and grass-fed red meat (e.g., lamb, beef, buffalo / bison)

- ✓ Organic and pasture-raised fowl (e.g., chicken, turkey)

Note: If you get most (or all) of your daily protein needs, predominantly from animal sources, then we recommend that you also include a variety of plant-based protein sources. This would be sustainable for your long-term health and that of our planet.

---

[44] It is not recommended for people who have (or had) cancer.

Appendix C: Healthy & Rich Sources of Fiber

Fruits	Vegetables	Nuts, Seeds, and Grains	Beans and Legumes
Avocado	Artichokes	Almonds	Black beans
Berries	Peas	Walnuts	Chick peas
Coconut	Okra	Flax	Lima beans
Pears	Winter squash	Chia	Split peas
Figs	Brussels sprouts	Quinoa	Lentils
Prunes	Cabbage	Oatmeal	Navy beans
Mango	Turnip	Barley	Pinto beans
Raisins	Broccoli	Bran flakes	
	Corn	Whole wheat	
	Carrots	Rye	
	Potato (with skin)	Wild rice	

Note: We recommend using organic sources whenever possible – to avoid harmful pesticides, herbicides, and genetically engineered ingredients.

Appendix D: Healthy Sources of Dietary Fats

Vegetarian, plant-based

- ✓ Avocado
- ✓ Nuts – walnuts, almonds, pistachios
- ✓ Seeds – sunflower, flax, chia
- ✓ Olives
- ✓ Dark chocolate[45]
- ✓ Coconut
- ✓ Organic soy – tofu, edamame
- ✓ Full-fat organic dairy (preferably raw or else pasteurized under low heat and non-homogenized)

Non-vegetarian, animal-based

- ✓ Pasture-raised organic eggs
- ✓ Wild caught fish – salmon, tuna[46]
- ✓ Grass-fed organic meats

Note: We recommend using organic sources whenever possible, especially soy products, animal meats, and dairy items that can contain genetically modified ingredients, if not certified organic.

---

[45] The higher the percentage (80% or more) of cocoa content, the lower the amount of added sugars / sweeteners.

[46] Eat sparingly due to higher mercury content compared to smaller fish.

Brief Testimonials

"Initially when I came to Nilanjana, I was experiencing very low energy and moods and was carrying extra weight. I was not really sure of how to eat or what foods were good for my body and I just felt down most of the time. I became aware of food's effects on my body and moods. I've learned so much about seasonal eating, the importance of a healthy gut and living more consciously in my life. I've started to work on meal planning which has helped our family. I am also bringing in more self care for myself, which has lifted my overall energy level and moods. What I especially love about working with Nilanjana is that we touch on so many areas of my life... It has been a wonderful holistic experience. I would recommend it to anyone who wants to get healthy in mind, body and spirit."

[N.E., age 45] Seattle, WA, USA

"I can't say enough good things about our sessions with Nilanjana. I approached her for weight loss and for overall wellbeing needs. My goal was to not only lose some weight, but have a healthier lifestyle in general. I was dealing with poor sleeping habits and stress - work related, relocating, etc.
During our sessions, I learned so much about how our bodies work, role of stress in our lives, and how to deal with all that not only by eating the right 'foods', also by incorporating meditation, herbal supplements, exercises, etc.
By the end, I was able to understand the role of nutrition in my life, use food as medicine, maintain a regular sleep schedule, find balance in every aspect of life and feel GREAT everyday!!
Even my kids now insist on eating organic, and they diligently read nutrition labels at the store."

[Priya, age 39] North Carolina, USA

"This is a much needed book, especially for busy professionals like me who have good intentions for a healthy lifestyle, but struggle to find simple practical steps toward that goal. I was a believer in quick fixes for health issues – until I had a gut-related one that surfaced as persistent burning skin rashes all over my body in 2011. I visited many doctors for a "magic pill" until every single one bailed out on me. I was in a quandary, playing victim and feeling terrible for months. The solution finally showed up in the form of a naturopath, once I came to terms with my situation and accepted it with a full heart. Being a skeptic about alternative medicine, I began consulting with the naturopath only because I did not have any other choice. To my surprise, she diagnosed my skin issue as gut-related, and

suggested a detox and a modified diet. My blood report indicated that I had to give up all the food items that were near and dear to me and were part of my staple. I was happy that there was a solution to my problem, but didn't have a clue how to get there. I was depressed and reached out to Nilanjana for help. She understood my issue, the naturopath's diagnosis and the food restrictions, and devised a meal plan that worked for me with minimal struggle. With her knowledge of organic food and other cooking ingredients, she offered me recipes that tasted the same but with healthier ingredients that were beneficial for me. To my awe, I healed over a course of six months – with no medication and minor changes in diet and lifestyle. Now, I am a firm believer in "food is medicine." I cannot thank her enough for being the miracle in my life.

I hope this book makes similar miracles happen in each and every reader's life."

[V.K., age 43] Seattle WA, USA

Index of Key Terms

omega-6 fatty acids 75-76, 79
omega-9 fatty acids 76
organic(ally) 53, 60, 62, 67, 69, 71-72, 75-76, 80-81, 86, 100, 125, 130, 136, 139-142

package(d) 15, 39, 79-80, 93, 111, 124
party 16, 118-119, 124-126
pasteurization 64-65, 68-69
personalized 4, 9, 47, 88, 98, 102, 123, 135
pesticide 19, 31-32, 34, 61, 81, 99, 100, 139, 141
plant(s) 25, 29, 32, 45-49, 52, 54-55, 64, 76, 93, 118, 140, 142
plastics 84, 101
poison 9-10, 33, 35, 54
prepared/preparation 15-16, 19, 27-30, 43, 47, 50, 57, 60, 63, 70, 79, 112, 124, 129-130, 133, 135
prescription: 3, 61, 86-87, 90, 136
preservative 32, 42, 83, 85, 103
prevention/preventative 3, 57-58, 64-65, 77, 137
price 20-21, 101, 107
principle(s) 1-3, 23-24, 28-29, 37, 40, 123, 136
processed 15-16, 25-26, 30-32, 38, 40-41, 48, 53-54, 56, 62-63, 65, 68-69, 71-72, 74, 76, 82, 85, 87, 90, 110-111, 118
production 2, 9, 20, 28, 46, 54, 64, 66-68, 70, 77, 83
protein 25, 27, 30, 35, 40, 45, 49, 50, 52-59, 64, 68-70, 86, 91, 93, 119, 140
pungent 35, 107

quality 1-2, 19, 21, 29, 31-32, 34, 47, 53, 55, 58, 60, 71, 80, 85-86, 92-93, 96, 98-100, 103
quantity 2, 16-17, 26, 33, 35-36, 41, 46, 49-50, 54, 65-67, 71, 93-94, 96-98

radiation 32, 86
rainbow 25-26
raw 2, 25, 30, 40-44, 69, 71, 75-76, 138, 142
rBGH/rBST 66-67, 69
reaction 24, 33, 51, 58-60
recalibrate 127-128
refine(d) 31-32, 65, 74
relationship 4, 11, 17, 33, 38, 107, 109, 121-122
resistance 40, 162
restaurant 15, 19, 80, 84, 86, 88, 111-112, 120
roadblock 114-116, 162

sabotage 114, 116
salt(y) 10, 32, 35, 46, 80, 82, 90, 98, 107, 110-111, 113
saturated fat 74-75, 77-78
school 16, 19, 28, 65, 78, 96, 120, 126, 132, 163
season 25, 27, 41-42, 61, 73, 129, 136
seed 29, 31, 47, 50, 57, 75-76, 91, 140, 142
self-discipline 88, 110
sensitive(ity) 24-25, 56, 59-60, 80, 115, 125
serving size 37, 39, 63, 93, 111, 124
signal 1, 10, 12, 16-17, 33, 90, 93-94, 97-98, 106-109, 128-129, 136
sleep 2, 40, 44, 77, 94, 96, 102, 104, 106, 121
soak(ing) 29, 43, 57, 60, 63, 96

150

References

The following references contain valid online links as of the date of this handbook's publication. Here, they are organized by the section, in which they appear in the handbook:

§ **Introduction:**
[Intro.1] *"108 Questions from the Secret Wisdom of Tibet", by Tulku Lama Lobsang* –
https://tulkulobsang.org/en/publications?layout=product&idProduct=121

§ **2:**
[2.1] *Health Benefits of Natural Foods* –
http://www.naturalfoodbenefits.com
[2.2] *Knowledge Is Power* –
http://www.thepowerhour.com/news2/healthy_food_chart.htm
[2.3] *Healing Food Reference* – http://www.healingfoodreference.com
[2.4] *"Yoga on Nutrition", by Omraam Mikhaël Aïvanhov* –
https://www.amazon.com/Yoga-Nutrition-Izvor-Collection-Book-ebook/dp/B00KOYPYRG/
[2.5] *The Grateful Brain – The Neuroscience of Giving Thanks* –
https://www.psychologytoday.com/blog/prefrontal-nudity/201211/the-grateful-brain
[2.6] *"Power vs. Force: The Hidden Determinants of Human Behavior", by Dr. David Hawkins* – https://www.amazon.com/Power-vs-Force-Determinants-Behavior-ebook/dp/B00EJBABS2/
[2.7] *Definition: Muscle Testing* –
http://www.selfgrowth.com/articles/definition_muscle_testing.html
[2.8] *Muscle Testing for Allergies* –
http://www.livestrong.com/article/199538-muscle-testing-for-allergies/
[2.9] *Which Method of Muscle Testing Is the Most Effective?* –
https://www.blissplan.com/mixed-bag/which-method-of-muscle-testing-is-the-most-effective/

§ **3:**
[3.1] *The W⁵H² Model* –
http://www.consultantsmind.com/2013/03/07/7-key-questions-who-what-why-when-where-how-how-much/
[3.2] *"Fountain of Youth Discovered", by Dr. Christiane Northrup* –
http://www.drnorthrup.com/fountain-of-youth-discovered-by-dr-northrup/

[3.3] *"Integrative Nutrition", by Joshua Rosenthal* –
https://www.amazon.com/Integrative-Nutrition-Third-Hunger-
Happiness-ebook/dp/B00IDEQGVC/

§ 4:
[4.1] *20 Diseases and Conditions Directly Attributable to Being
Overweight* –
http://articles.mercola.com/sites/articles/archive/2008/09/02/20-
diseases-and-conditions-directly-attributable-to-being-overweight.aspx

§ 5:
[5.1] *"Ayurveda: The Science of Self-Healing – A Practical Guide", by
Dr. Vasant Lad* – https://www.amazon.com/Ayurveda-Science-Healing-
Practical-Guide/dp/0914955004/
[5.2] *Metabolic Typing* –
http://www.themetabolicinstitute.com/MetabolicTyping.htm
[5.3] *"The Metabolic Typing Diet", by William Wolcott and Trish
Fahey* – http://www.metabolictypingdiet.com
[5.4] *The Blood Type Diet* – http://www.dadamo.com
[5.5] *Body Type Quiz* – http://lifespa.com/ayurvedic-health-
quizzes/body-type-quiz/
[5.6] *Healthy Eating Rainbow Fruits and Vegetables Text Poster* –
http://www.zazzle.com/healthy_eating_rainbow_fruits_and_vegetables_te
xt_poster-228784320869275825
[5.7] *What Are Hypoallergenic Foods? An Overview of Low
Allergenicity Foods* – http://healwithfood.org/articles/what-are-
hypoallergenic-foods.php
[5.8] *Sneezy, Drippy? Don't Be Dopey!* – https://lifespa.com/sneezy-
drippy-dont-dopey/
[5.9] *The Confusing World of Eating, Dieting, and Cleansing* –
https://lifespa.com/confusing-world-of-eating-dieting-and-cleansing/

§ 6:
[6.1] *The pH Miracle – Alkaline-Acid Food Chart* –
http://www.phmiracleliving.com/t-food-chart.aspx
[6.2] *High-Temperature Cooking & The World's Healthiest Foods* –
http://www.whfoods.com/genpage.php?tname=george&dbid=122
[6.3] *The Hidden Hazards of Microwave Cooking* –
https://www.health-science.com/microwave_hazards.html

[6.4] *"Choosing the Right Cooking Oil", PCC Natural Markets* – http://www.pccnaturalmarkets.com/products/grocery/Cooking-Oil-Brochure-062414.pdf

[6.5] *"Cultured Food for Life – How to Make and Serve Delicious Probiotic Foods for Better Health and Wellness", by Donna Schwenk* – https://www.amazon.com/Cultured-Food-Life-Delicious-Probiotic/dp/1401942822/

[6.6] *"Energetics of Food", by Steve Gagne* – https://static-learn.integrativenutrition.com/cdn/farfuture/6Pi4rdPuaVZVaqYHRgyNZ8u0vN7SEdjbZ4yZ25Gw5yA/mtime:1437590565/sites/default/files/slides/The%20Energetics%20of%20Food%20Swith%20Steve%20Gagne%20Slides_July15.pdf?view=FitV

[6.7] *Energetics* – https://en.wikipedia.org/wiki/Energetics

[6.8] *"Food Energetics – The Spiritual, Emotional, and Nutritional Power of What We Eat", by Steve Gagne* – https://www.amazon.com/Food-Energetics-Spiritual-Emotional-Nutritional/dp/1594772428/

§ 7:

[7.1] *Playing God in the Garden* – http://michaelpollan.com/articles-archive/playing-god-in-the-garden/

[7.2] *Chemical Used in Non-Stick Cookware Continues to Prove Its Toxicity* – http://www.naturalnews.com/022645.html

[7.3] *Adverse Effects of Chemical Fertilizers and Pesticides on Human Health and Environment* – http://www.jchps.com/specialissues/Special%20issue3/34%20jchps%20si3%20addn%20K.Anitha%20Kumari%20150-151.pdf

[7.4] *A Review of the Science on the Potential Health Effects of Pesticide Residues on Food and Related Statements Made by Interest Groups* – http://www.safefruitsandveggies.com/sites/default/files/expert-panel-report.pdf

[7.5] *Pesticides – Children's Health and the Environment* – http://www.who.int/ceh/capacity/Pesticides.pdf

[7.6] *Health Risks* – http://responsibletechnology.org/gmo-education/health-risks/

[7.7] *GM Foods More Dangerous for Children Than Adults* – http://articles.mercola.com/sites/articles/archive/2010/10/07/gm-foods-more-dangerous-for-children-than-adults.aspx

[7.8] *"Millions against Monsanto"* and *"GMO No"* – https://www.organicconsumers.org/sites/default/files/gmo-no.pdf

[7.9] *Non-GMO Shopping Guide* – http://nongmoshoppingguide.com

§ 8:

[8.1] *FAQs – Mesopotamia through Shakespeare –* http://www.foodtimeline.org/foodfaq3.html

[8.2] *Why Did We Evolve a Taste for Sweetness? –* http://perfecthealthdiet.com/2011/03/why-did-we-evolve-a-taste-for-sweetness/

[8.3] *Sweet Taste Preferences Are Partly Genetically Determined –* http://ajcn.nutrition.org/content/86/1/55.full

[8.4] *The History of Sweeteners –* http://www.hermesetas.com/data/en/specialised/sweeteners/history.php

[8.5] *Sweet Poison: How Sugar, Not Cocaine, Is One of the Most Addictive and Dangerous Substances –* http://www.nydailynews.com/life-style/health/white-poison-danger-sugar-beat-article-1.1605232

[8.6] *"Sugar: The Bitter Truth", by UCTV –* https://www.youtube.com/watch?v=dBnniua6-oM

[8.7] *The Bitter Truth about Sugar –* http://articles.mercola.com/sites/articles/archive/2014/12/31/bitter-truth-sugar.aspx

[8.8] *Comprehensive Information about Sugar and Sweeteners of All Types –* http://www.sugar-and-sweetener-guide.com

[8.9] *How High-Sugar Diets Speed You toward an Early Grave –* http://articles.mercola.com/sites/articles/archive/2016/09/07/recommended-sugar-intake.aspx

[8.10] *The Sugar and Cancer Connection: Why Sugar is Called "The White Death" –* https://thetruthaboutcancer.com/sugar-white-death/

[8.11] *"Integrative Nutrition", by Joshua Rosenthal –* https://www.amazon.com/Integrative-Nutrition-Third-Hunger-Happiness-ebook/dp/B00IDEQGVC/

§ 9:

[9.1] *"Is Sugar Toxic", by Gary Taubes –* http://www.nytimes.com/2011/04/17/magazine/mag-17Sugar-t.html

[9.2] *"Blood Sugar: Your Key to Vibrant Health – Tips for Lowering Your Blood Sugar Naturally", by Dr. Christiane Northrup –* http://www.drnorthrup.com/blood-sugar-your-key-to-vibrant-health/

[9.3] *"Women's Bodies, Women's Wisdom: Creating Physical and Emotional Health and Healing", by Dr. Christiane Northrup –* https://www.amazon.com/Womens-Bodies-Wisdom-Revised-Emotional/dp/0553386735/

[9.4] *"Inner Engineering – A Yogi's Guide to Joy"*, *by Sadhguru* –
https://www.amazon.com/Inner-Engineering-Yogis-Guide-
Joy/dp/0143428845/

[9.5] *"The Miracle of Fasting: Proven throughout History for Physical,
Mental, & Spiritual Rejuvenation"*, *by Patricia Bragg and Paul C.
Bragg* – http://bragg.com/books/mof_excerpt.html

[9.6] *"Eating Well for Optimum Health"*, *by Andrew Weil, M.D.* –
https://www.amazon.com/Eating-Well-Optimum-Health-
Essential/dp/0060959584/

§ 10:

[10.1] *Food Webs and Bioaccumulation* –
https://www.nwf.org/Wildlife/Wildlife-Conservation/Food-Webs.aspx

[10.2] *"Inner Engineering – A Yogi's Guide to Joy" (p. 136), by
Sadhguru* – https://www.amazon.com/Inner-Engineering-Yogis-Guide-
Joy/dp/0143428845/

§ 11:

[11.1] *Dr. Russell Blaylock Interviewed for "The Truth about Cancer"
(episode 4)* –
https://www.facebook.com/thetruthaboutcancer/posts/100569940952336
8

[11.2] *Complete Protein: How Much and What Kind to Eat* –
http://lifespa.com/complete-protein-much-kind-eat/

[11.3] *Vegetarian Protein Foods* –
http://www.nomeatathlete.com/vegetarian-protein/

[11.4] *Bad News for Factory Farming* –
http://articles.mercola.com/sites/articles/archive/2016/07/06/factory-
farming-cafos-foodborne-illnesses.aspx

[11.5] *American Meat – An Inside Look at Sustainable Farming in
America* –
http://articles.mercola.com/sites/articles/archive/2013/11/23/american-
meat.aspx

[11.6] *Is Organic Better for Your Health? A Look at Milk, Meat, Eggs,
Produce, and Fish* – https://www.washingtonpost.com/national/health-
science/is-organic-better-for-your-health-a-look-at-milk-meat-eggs-
produce-and-fish/2014/04/07/036c654e-a313-11e3-8466-
d34c451760b9_story.html

[11.7] *The Protein Myth: Why You Need Less Protein Than You
Think* – http://www.huffingtonpost.com/jessica-jones-ms-rd/protein-
diet_b_1882372.html

[11.8] *Protein Chart* – http://www.lose-weight-with-us.com/list-of-high-protein-foods.html

[11.9] *The Basics Made Simple* – http://buildhealthykids.com/basics.html

[11.10] *"Advanced Pranic Healing: The Most Advanced Energy Healing System Using Color Pranas", by Master Choa Kok Sui* – https://www.amazon.com/Advanced-Pranic-Healing-Latest-Secrets/dp/B0049POHM4/

[11.11] *Blood Type 'O'* – http://www.dadamo.com/txt/index.pl?1004

[11.12] *10 Reasons Why the Meat and Dairy Industry Is Unsustainable* – http://www.care2.com/causes/10-reasons-why-the-meat-and-dairy-industry-is-unsustainable.html

§ 12:

[12.1] *The 10 Most Important Crops in the World* – http://www.businessinsider.com/10-crops-that-feed-the-world-2011-9#2-wheat-9

[12.2] *The 4 Reasons Why I Switched to Einkorn Wheat* – http://www.thehealthyhomeeconomist.com/the-4-reasons-why-im-switching-to-einkorn-wheat/

[12.3] *Einkorn: The Staff of Life That Wheat Once Was* – http://www.amaluxherbal.com/einkorn-staff-life-wheat/

[12.4] *All about Lectins: Here's What You Need to Know* – http://www.precisionnutrition.com/all-about-lectins

[12.5] *Ask JJ: Lectins and Phytates* – http://www.huffingtonpost.com/jj-virgin/ask-jj-lectins-and-phytat_b_9623754.html

[12.6] *The Little Known Secrets about Bleached Flour* – http://articles.mercola.com/sites/articles/archive/2009/03/26/The-Little-Known-Secrets-about-Bleached-Flour.aspx

[12.7] *6 Reasons Why Gluten Is Bad for Some People* – https://authoritynutrition.com/6-shocking-reasons-why-gluten-is-bad/

[12.8] *Dr. William Davis, Gluten Summit 2013* – http://www.theglutensummit.com/

[12.9] *Loren Cordain, Gluten Summit 2013* – http://www.theglutensummit.com/

[12.10] *Dr. Alessio Fasano, Gluten Summit 2013* – http://www.theglutensummit.com/

[12.11] *Gluten Free? What to Do If You "Get Glutened"* – http://avivaromm.com/what-to-do-if-you-get-glutened/#

[12.12] *Dr. John Douillard* – http://www.lifespa.com

[12.13] *5 Unexpected Sources of Gluten That Are Not Food* –
http://www.huffingtonpost.com/2013/09/07/non-food-gluten-products-
sources_n_3791886.html

§ 13:
[13.1] *Neolithic Revolution* –
https://en.wikipedia.org/wiki/Neolithic_Revolution
[13.2] *Industrial Revolution* –
https://en.wikipedia.org/wiki/Industrial_Revolution
[13.3] *Louis Pasteur* – https://en.wikipedia.org/wiki/Louis_Pasteur
[13.4] *All about the Dairy Group* –
https://www.choosemyplate.gov/dairy
[13.5] *Turns out Your "Hormone-Free" Milk Is Full of Sex Hormones* –
http://www.motherjones.com/media/2014/04/milk-hormones-cancer-
pregnant-cows-estrogen
[13.6] *Bovine Growth Hormone: Milk Does Nobody Good* –
http://www.ejnet.org/bgh/nogood.html
[13.7] *The Dangers of Drinking Cow's Milk* –
http://www.globalhealingcenter.com/natural-health/dangers-of-cows-
milk/
[13.8] *Dangers of Pasteurization and Homogenization* –
http://preventdisease.com/news/10/111810_dangers_pasteurization_hom
ogenization.shtml
[13.9] *Is It Healthier to Drink Grass-Fed or Organic Milk?* –
http://www.theglobeandmail.com/life/health-and-fitness/health/is-it-
healthier-to-drink-grass-fed-or-organic-milk/article20726402/
[13.10] *Health Benefits of Organic vs. Conventional Milk* –
http://articles.mercola.com/sites/articles/archive/2014/01/14/conventio
nal-vs-organic-milk.aspx
[13.11] *15 Amazing Benefits of Ghee* –
http://www.care2.com/greenliving/15-amazing-benefits-of-ghee.html
[13.12] *Goat Milk Benefits Are Superior to Cow Milk* –
https://draxe.com/goat-milk/
[13.13] *Health Benefits of Sheep Milk* –
http://beveragesandhealth.com/health-benefits-of-sheep-milk/

§ 14:
[14.1] *6 Graphs that Show Why the "War" on Fat Was a Huge
Mistake* – https://authoritynutrition.com/6-graphs-the-war-on-fat-was-a-
mistake/

[14.2] *Diet Mythology: Ancel Keys and the Fat Fallacy* –
http://www.leangains.com/2010/06/diet-mythology-ancel-keys-fat-
fallacy.html

[14.3] *Time Magazine: We Were Wrong about Saturated Fats* –
http://healthimpactnews.com/2014/time-magazine-we-were-wrong-about-
saturated-fats/

[14.4] *An Epic Debunking of the Saturated Fat Myth* –
https://authoritynutrition.com/it-aint-the-fat-people/

[14.5] *Omega-3, -6, -9 Health Benefits and Sources* – http://wiki-
fitness.com/omega-3-6-9-health-benefits-and-sources/

[14.6] *Fats: Why Healthy Dietary Fat Is Crucial* –
http://www.mercola.com/nutritionplan/beginner_fats.htm

[14.7] *New Science Destroys the Saturated Fat Myth* –
http://articles.mercola.com/sites/articles/archive/2014/07/27/saturated-
fat-cholesterol.aspx#

[14.8] *Understanding Cholesterol Numbers* –
http://www.webmd.com/cholesterol-management/guide/understanding-
numbers#1

[14.9] *How to Make Sense of Your Cholesterol Levels Infographic* –
http://www.mercola.com/infographics/cholesterol-levels.htm

[14.10] *Why I Believe Over Half of Your Diet Should Be Made up of
Saturated Fat* –
http://articles.mercola.com/sites/articles/archive/2012/05/31/coconut-
oil-for-healthy-heart.aspx

[14.11] *Fatty-Acid Metabolism Disorder* –
https://en.wikipedia.org/wiki/Fatty-acid_metabolism_disorder

§ 15:

[15.1] *Nutrition Facts Label* –
http://www.fda.gov/downloads/Food/IngredientsPackagingLabeling/Lab
elingNutrition/UCM272926.pdf

[15.2] *Guidance for Industry: A Food Labeling Guide* –
http://www.fda.gov/Food/GuidanceRegulation/GuidanceDocumentsReg
ulatoryInformation/LabelingNutrition/ucm064880.htm#ingredient

[15.3] *"Dirty Dozen"* –
https://www.ewg.org/foodnews/dirty_dozen_list.php

[15.4] *"Clean Fifteen"* –
https://www.ewg.org/foodnews/clean_fifteen_list.php

[15.5] *11 Food Ingredients Banned outside the U.S. That We Eat* –
http://abcnews.go.com/Lifestyle/Food/11-foods-banned-
us/story?id=19457237

[15.6] *24 Potentially Harmful Food Additives* –
http://www.wereyouwondering.com/possible-and-suspected-carcinogens-found-in-food

[15.7] *List of the More Widely Known Dangerous Ingredients in Body and Food Products* –
http://www.purezing.com/living/toxins/living_toxins_dangerousingredients.html

[15.8] *How Food Companies Exploit Americans with Ingredients Banned in Other Countries* – http://foodbabe.com/tag/ingredients-banned-in-other-countries/

[15.9] *Common Plastics #1 to #7* –
https://www.lifewithoutplastic.com/store/common_plastics_no_1_to_no_7

§ 16:

[16.1] *85 Snack Ideas for Kids and Adults* –
http://www.100daysofrealfood.com/2012/07/31/85-snacks-for-kids-and-adults/

§ 17:

[17.1] *"Human Longevity: Genetics or Lifestyle? It Takes Two to Tango", by Giuseppe Passarino, Francesco De Rango, and Alberto Montesanto* –
http://immunityageing.biomedcentral.com/articles/10.1186/s12979-016-0066-z

[17.2] *Live with the Natural Cycles* – https://lifespa.com/live-with-the-cycles/

[17.3] *"Eating Well for Optimum Health", by Dr. Andrew Weill* –
https://www.amazon.com/Eating-Well-Optimum-Health-Essential/dp/0525431799/

§ 18:

[18.1] *"The Power of Water", by Sadhguru* –
https://www.innerengineering.com/online/blog/the-power-of-water

[18.2] *What Percent of Earth is Water?* –
http://www.universetoday.com/65588/what-percent-of-earth-is-water/

[18.3] *"Water: The Shocking Truth That Can Save Your Life", by Patricia Bragg* – https://www.amazon.com/Water-Shocking-Truth-That-Save/dp/0877900655

[18.4] *Be Like Water* –
http://www.creationsmagazine.com/articles/C115/Dyer.html

[18.5] *The Best Water Filter Systems* –
http://www.toptenreviews.com/health/wellness/best-water-filter-systems/

[18.6] *4 Ways to Remove Fluoride and Other Harmful Chemicals from Your Water* – http://readynutrition.com/resources/4-ways-to-remove-fluoride-and-other-harmful-chemicals-from-your-water_18032015/

[18.7] *How to Make Alkaline Water at Home* –
http://www.alkalinebenefits.net/how-to-make-alkaline-water-for-drinking/

[18.8] *How to Make Your Own Alkaline Water at Home* –
http://www.youngandraw.com/how-to-make-your-own-alkaline-water-at-home-2/

[18.9] *Structured Water – an Interview with Dr. Gerald Pollack* –
http://articles.mercola.com/sites/articles/archive/2011/01/29/dr-pollack-on-structured-water.aspx

[18.10] *"The Healing Power of Water", by Dr. Masaru Emoto* –
https://www.amazon.com/Healing-Power-Water-Masaru-Emoto/dp/1401908772/

[18.11] *"The Water Wizard: The Extraordinary Power of Natural Water", by Viktor Schauberger* – https://www.amazon.com/Water-Wizard-Extraordinary-Properties-Natural/dp/1858600480

[18.12] *"The Fourth Phase of Water: Beyond Solid, Liquid, and Vapor", by Dr. Gerald Pollack* – https://www.amazon.com/Fourth-Phase-Water-Beyond-Liquid/dp/0962689548

[18.13] *"The Fourth Phase of Water", by Dr. Gerald Pollack* –
https://www.westonaprice.org/health-topics/health-issues/the-fourth-phase-of-water/

[18.14] *Safe Cosmetics* – http://www.safecosmetics.org/

§ 19:

[19.1] *"My Incredible Talking Body", by Rebecca Bowen* –
https://www.amazon.com/Incredible-Talking-Body-Rebecca-Bowen/dp/0997196203/

[19.2] *"Heal Your Body", by Louise Hay* –
https://www.amazon.com/Heal-Your-Body-Louise-Hay/dp/0937611352

[19.3] *"Mirror Work: 21 Days to Heal Your Life", by Louise Hay* –
http://www.hayhouse.com/mirror-work-paperback

[19.4] *The Neuroscience of Mindfulness Meditation* –
http://www.chopra.com/articles/the-neuroscience-of-mindfulness-meditation

[19.5] *Aikido and the Taming of the Reptilian Brain* –
http://aikidojournal.com/2016/06/29/aikido-and-the-taming-of-the-reptilian-brain-by-stanley-pranin/

[19.6] *Can Martial Arts Help Children with ADHD Focus?* –
http://www.healthcentral.com/adhd/c/1443/134526/martial-children-adhd/

§ 20:

[20.1] *Physiology of Taste* –
http://www.vivo.colostate.edu/hbooks/pathphys/digestion/pregastric/taste.html

[20.2] *The Flavorists: Tweaking Taste and Creating Cravings* –
http://www.cbsnews.com/news/the-flavorists-tweaking-tastes-and-creating-cravings-27-11-2011/

[20.3] *Slideshow: High Sodium Shockers* –
http://www.webmd.com/diet/ss/slideshow-salt-shockers

[20.4] *Health Benefits of Natural Foods* –
http://www.naturalfoodbenefits.com

[20.5] *The 25 Unhealthiest Junk Food Items* –
http://kimberlysnyder.com/blog/2012/02/28/the-25-unhealthiest-junk-food-items/

§ 21:

[21.1] *"The Big Leap", by Gay Hendricks* –
https://www.amazon.com/Big-Leap-Conquer-Hidden-Level-ebook/dp/B0026772QU/

[21.2] *"Mastery: The Keys to Success and Long-Term Fulfillment", by George Leonard* – https://www.amazon.com/dp/B01ND0X91Y/

§ 24:

[24.1] *27 Healthy and Portable High-Protein Snacks* –
http://greatist.com/health/high-protein-snacks-portable

[24.2] *10 Quick Make-Ahead Snack Ideas for Food Prep Day* –
http://www.organizeyourselfskinny.com/2015/05/27/10-quick-make-ahead-snack-ideas-for-food-prep-day/

About the Authors

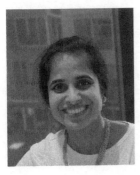

Nilanjana Krishnan is a certified Integrative Nutrition Health Coach, founder of "Wellness with Nilanjana, LLC," and a published author. Her mission is to inspire and empower nurturers, like herself, to become inspiring role models – especially for children – by creating a life of their dreams through conscious living strategies, harmonizing their physical, mental, emotional, and spiritual health. Nilanjana uses a holistic approach, personalized for each client, to help them: (a) identify and clarify their intentions with respect to health and other important life goals; (b) eliminate – or reduce the impact of – roadblocks or resistances they may experience; (c) achieve optimum health of body, mind, and spirit; and (d) be empowered to move confidently in the direction of their dreams, experiencing the life they envision.

Her previous book, "I Know The Way – 81 fun ways to live the Tao" is a family friendly, experiential learning tool that includes fables, words of wisdom, and affirmations to help reinforce the deeper teachings.

Nilanjana has also graduated from the "Life Education Program" offered by the CwG Foundation, under the mentorship of Neale Donald Walsch, a contemporary spiritual teacher and New York Times bestselling author. Her formal education includes a Bachelors degree in Electronics Engineering from Anna University in Chennai, India, and a Masters in Business Administration from Southern New Hampshire University. She is also a Reiki energy-healing practitioner.

She lives in the Greater Seattle area with her husband and their two young boys. Nilanjana enjoys cooking, yoga, meditation, music, and dance-based fitness routines.

She can be contacted at HealthCoachNilanjana@gmail.com and also via www.WellnessWithNilanjana.com and www.facebook.com/nilanjana.krishnan.

162

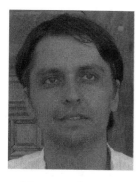**Valentin Razmov** is an award-winning teacher, a holistic coach, an author, and a certified yoga instructor. After moving to the United States to deepen his education, he found his calling in spreading messages of empowerment and inspiring others to reach beyond what they believe to be possible. Today, his passion leads him to regularly engage in creative and unconventional ways with audiences of all ages in a variety of subjects and settings – from leadership and software project management at the university level; to chess and analytical thinking in schools and online; to conscious living, nutrition, and holistic wellbeing with children and their caretakers; to yoga and meditation at spiritual centers and in college classrooms.

The results have been transformative to many. Deeper insights about life and the interdependence of everything; wisdom from world spiritual traditions; and a calm, pragmatic, and balanced attitude even in the face of difficult challenges. A number of his students find ways to come back for more.

Valentin has authored many scientific papers, and also co-authored a textbook for junior software engineers. He holds a Ph.D. in Computer Science & Engineering from the University of Washington, Seattle, and a Master's degree in that discipline from Sofia University in Bulgaria.

He is a Pranic Healing practitioner and a student of great spiritual masters, including Master Choa Kok Sui, Sadhguru Jaggi Vasudev, and Paramhansa Yogananda. He finds deep fulfillment to be of service.

Valentin lives in the Greater Seattle area with his wife and their two children. He is inspired by music, loves the outdoors, practices several styles of yoga and meditation, and enjoys stretching his mind with thoughtful books and conversations.

He can be contacted at VRazmov@gmail.com. You can also find him on LinkedIn: www.LinkedIn.com/in/VRazmov.

57283346R00098

Made in the USA
San Bernardino, CA
18 November 2017